An Autobibliography by John Caius

John Caius (1510–1573), second founder of Gonville and Caius College, Cambridge, was an English scholar with an international reputation in his lifetime as a naturalist, historian and medical writer. His *Autobibliography* is a major contribution to the history of English culture in the middle years of the sixteenth century and has been translated into English for the first time in this book.

Beginning with an in-depth introduction to John Caius' life and works, *An Autobibliography by John Caius* provides a wealth of information to support and accompany the translation of this significant text. In his *Autobibliography*, Caius lists the books that he wrote but also details the circumstances of their writing. He describes his travels in Italy in search of manuscripts of the ancient Greek doctor Galen of Pergamum as well as giving an insight into his personal life, including his vigorously conservative views, whether on medicine, spelling and pronunciation, or on Cambridge University. His religious views, which led to the ransacking of his rooms by a Cambridge mob, are explored in detail in Appendix II of this book. In Appendix I, recent discoveries of books owned and annotated by Caius are used to supplement what he says about his activities, as well as to trace at least one of his lost works in Italy and Denmark.

The resulting picture throws light on European medicine in the sixteenth century, as well as on the humanistic culture that linked learned men and women across Renaissance Europe.

Vivian Nutton is Professor of the History of Medicine, I.M. Sechenov First Moscow State Medical University, and Emeritus Professor of the History of Medicine, University College London. Among his recent books are a translation of Galen, *On Distress* (2013), *Ancient Medicine*, 2ed (2013), and a translation of Johann Guinter and Andreas Vesalius, *Principles of Anatomy according to the Opinion of Galen* (2017).

Routledge Early Modern Translations

In the same series:

Principles of Anatomy according to the Opinion of Galen by Johann Guinter and Andreas Vesalius
Edited by Vivian Nutton

An Autobibliography **by John Caius**
Edited by Vivian Nutton

An Autobibliography
by John Caius

Edited by Vivian Nutton

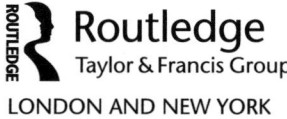
Routledge
Taylor & Francis Group

LONDON AND NEW YORK

First published 2018 by Routledge
2 Park Square, Milton Park, Abingdon, Oxon OX14 4RN

and by Routledge
605 Third Avenue, New York, NY 10017

First issued in paperback 2021

Routledge is an imprint of the Taylor & Francis Group, an informa business

British Library Cataloguing-in-Publication Data
A catalogue record for this book is available from the British Library

Library of Congress Cataloging-in-Publication Data
Names: Caius, John, 1510–1573, author. | Nutton, Vivian, editor.
Title: An autobibliography / by John Caius ; edited by Vivian Nutton.
   Other titles: De libris propriis. English
Description: Abingdon, Oxon ; New York, NY : Routledge, 2018. |
   Series: Microhistories | Includes bibliographical references and index.
Identifiers: LCCN 2018001028 | ISBN 9781138069121 (hardback : alk.
   paper) | ISBN 9781315157320 (ebook)
Subjects: LCSH: Caius, John, 1510–1573. | Medicine—Europe—
   History—16th century. | Humanism—Europe—History—16th century. |
   Physicians—Great Britain—Biography. | Scholars—Great Britain—
   Biography.
Classification: LCC R489.C3 C35 2018 | DDC 610.94—dc23
LC record available at https://lccn.loc.gov/2018001028

ISBN 13: 978-1-03-209529-5 (pbk)
ISBN 13: 978-1-138-06912-1 (hbk)

Typeset in Times New Roman
by Apex CoVantage, LLC

**To my Cambridge teachers and friends
over more than half a century**

Contents

Figures

Acknowledgements

My first debt is to three distinguished and now-deceased fellows of Gonville and Caius College, Charles Brink, Philip Grierson and Christopher Brooke, who encouraged this non-Caian thirty years ago to become interested in the second founder of their college. Indeed, I was fortunate to be able more recently to discuss some of the problems raised in this book with Christopher Brooke, as well as with two other fellows, Michael Prichard and Richard Duncan-Jones. Another Cambridge friend, Michael Reeve, has been always helpful in dealing with the complexities of Caius' Latin, and greatly encouraged me in the researches into Caius' work on Galen that I published in 1987. But although much of this book is concerned with Galen and with manuscripts in distant libraries, it must be understood against a much wider background of humanist studies in Britain and elsewhere. Caius was a polymath, and a translator has frequently to rely on the expertise of others, generously given, to understand fully the significance of many of his observations. Over the years I have been fortunate to be able to retrace many of Caius' steps and to visit many of the Italian institutions mentioned by him, most notably at Padua, where I have been the guest at meetings organised by Silvia Ferretto, Pietro Gori, Maurizio Rippa-Bonati, Massimo Rinaldi and Gaetano Thiene. Fabio Zampieri helped resolve some of my Paduan queries, and Fabiola Zurlini has been extraordinarily diligent in securing for me copies of rare Italian publications. My understanding of Caius' anatomical studies has been much helped by discussions with Francis Van Glabbeek and Julius Rocca. The two appendices resulted from questions asked by friends. Andrew Burnett's find of a reference to Caius in an Oxford note led me to the rediscovery of some of Caius' conclusions he had written in a work now lost. I am grateful also for their help in tracing the fate of this book, and of others that were never published, to Nils Bruun, Klaus-Dietrich Fisher, Clarine Rijpstra-Van Daal, Sergio Sconocchia and Anders Toftgaard. My interest in Tudor Cambridge, stimulated half a century ago by discussions with the late Harry Porter, has been much refined through the assistance of Ceri Law, who showed me chapters in her forthcoming book, and of Diarmaid MacCulloch, who commented critically on a draft of the appendix. I have also benefited from conversations and correspondence with Elisa Andretti, Fabrizio Bigotti,

Katharine Craik, Peter Godman, Paul Gwynne, Urs Leu, Grantley MacDonald, Richard Smith, Andrew Wear and Barbara Zipser, as well as from the genial assistance of librarians at the British Library, the Cambridge University Library, the Classical Institute, London, Eton College, Gonville and Caius College, the Wellcome Library and that great repository of European values, the Warburg Institute. The book's referees provided helpful advice as well as some salutary corrections. Claudia Stein read a draft of the book, as did Holger Funk, who provided me with much material on Conrad Gessner that would otherwise have been unknown to me. Florike Egmond kindly entertained me in Rome and allowed me to see her reproductions of Caius' and Gessner's pictures in Amsterdam. My wife, as always, read the manuscript and improved both its English and its argument, and my granddaughter, Saskia Oswald, helped with the index. The editorial staff at Routledge have been their usual helpful selves. To all of them I am most grateful; any errors that remain are entirely my own. Reviewers will decide whether the book lives up to the standards (or to use a favourite word of John Caius, the *virtus*) of the scholar whose life and works are described within it.

Part I
Introduction

Preface

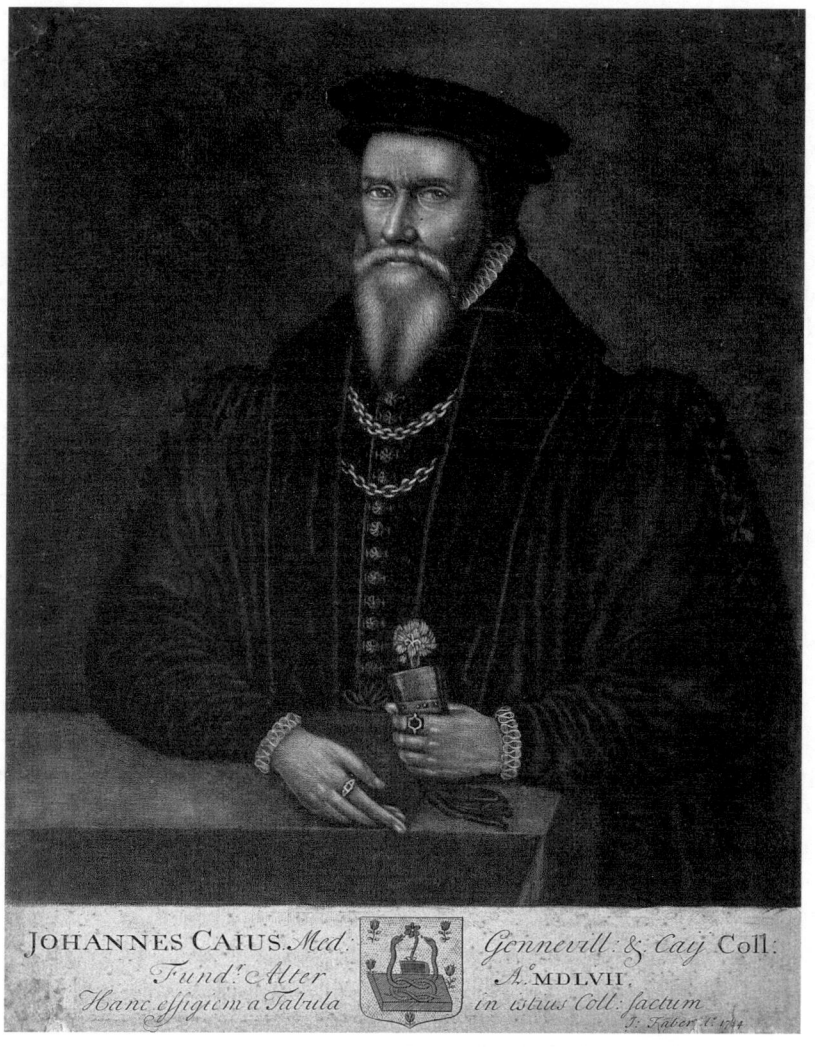

Figure 1 John Caius (1510–1573). Mezzotint by J. Faber, 1650.

John Caius' autobibliography, *De libris suis/De libris propriis, An Autobib-liography*, is a remarkable document that has not received the attention that it deserves. First published in 1570 as the last work in a volume concerned more with natural history, it was reprinted with corrections in 1729, and again in 1912 in the volume of his works edited by E. S. Roberts, Master of Gonville and Caius College, to celebrate the 400th anniversary of his birth. Samuel Jebb, the editor of the 1729 edition, thought it important not to for-get his achievements, especially as they showed the vigour of the Classical Tradition within medicine, and most notably at the College of Physicians of London.[1] But compared to his other tracts, it seems to have been little read, and in an increasingly Latin-less age, its complex High Renaissance Latin adds a further obstacle to understanding its message. Nor has it always been well served by its admirers. John Venn, whose detailed biography prefaces Roberts' edition, described it simply as 'a minute account of his writings, both published and unpublished', a description that is partially misleading and hardly likely to attract readers who lack an interest in bibliography. With greater justice, another devoted Caian, Philip Grierson, declared in his intro-duction to the inventory of Caius' library that it was 'one of those tantalizing works that never tell one quite enough'. It is true that it deliberately leaves out or abridges large parts of Caius' life, most notably the refounding of his Cam-bridge College and his activities at the London College of Physicians, which can be reconstructed from other sources and from what he wrote elsewhere, but these local initiatives were, in Caius' view, secondary to the importance of his publications on the international stage. Nor does this treatise fit easily into the history of autobiography, in part because its self-fashioning is not as obvious as in many other medical lives. Besides, Caius was no Erasmus, no Thomas More, and the life of a scholar does not hold out much promise of excitement. His conservatism and, until very recently, the denigration of the standard medical theories of his age as outdated and dangerous to patients, deterred medical historians from investigating his life and writings further. His religious views and the catastrophe of his last months also diverted his-torians until very recently from setting him in his proper Cambridge context of the 1560s and 1570s.

Such neglect can now hardly be justified, as a variety of studies over the past two decades has shown. In this book, which crosses the boundaries of genre, Caius provides information on his life and early career that illu-minates a period in English intellectual life marked by the spread of Euro-pean ideas on humanism, and especially on humanism within medicine. The rediscovery of texts from classical antiquity that had been lost for centuries gave authority to those, like Caius, who revered the past and who often saw in them progress over their medieval successors. The recovery of Galen in his original Greek from the 1470s onward provided doctors of the Renais-sance with an abundance of new material on therapeutics and, in particular, anatomy that proved inspirational. The book's digressions, polemics and repetitions also allow a reconstruction of the influential Cambridge figure that others would have known and Caius wished to project. New findings, most notably of the private information contained in Caius' own annotated copies of Galen and other volumes in his library, complement this public description of his activities and help to place him within a wider European context. He is a British writer of the Elizabethan period who is unusual in being published several times abroad and in enjoying an international reputation for his scholarship in medicine and in natural history. This short text is also a lament for the past at a point in English history when such nostalgia was frowned upon by others more progressive, and when the centuries-old synthesis of Galenic medicine was beginning to be challenged by new ideas (although it took more than three centuries before it was entirely abandoned). But to view this book in the light of what was yet to come, as has often been done, is to misunderstand much of what Caius was trying to do. As will become clear in the notes and appendices to this translation, he was far from being alone in his opinions, and he shared his intellectual interests with many leading scholars of his day.

A renaissance commentator, Filippo Beroaldo the elder (1453–1505), described the duty of commentators as being to unravel meanings, explain obscurities and uncover secrets in a chosen author.[2] They should in consequence be honoured for diligently and meticulously untying any knots and for benefiting posterity by their night vigils. Beroaldo was speaking about the obscurities of the Latin poet Propertius, but his remarks apply equally well to those of John Caius. Like his hero Galen of Pergamum, Caius was a polymath. The wide-ranging nature of his publications, and the topics he chose to include in this tract, present enormous problems to any commentator. Caius' Latin, as befits a Cambridge don, is extremely learned and allusive, and his classical references are both copious and recondite. Not all have been identified, or can be easily recognised in an English translation, and I have noted only a few of Caius' most obvious or most surprising sources, but his contemporaries would have appreciated their range and the elegance with which they were deployed. Caius was also a doctor, working in a framework of ideas and explanations that are not those of today, as well as an Englishman living, working and travelling in Europe at a particular historical juncture as confessional differences began to harden, and adherence to the old ways could prove as dangerous, and on occasions as deadly, as a passion for innovation. A generation earlier or later, Caius would have had different priorities and different chances of success. But above all, he was a European scholar, with links across Europe and with interests that were widely shared. To recreate that humanist universe is a major task for any editor, not least because relevant material may not be easy to hand or even all located in one major library. The growing tendency of British libraries over the last decades not to purchase books in languages other than English also inhibits access to Continental scholarship, and not just to the more local publications. This insularity is partly balanced by the increasing availability of sixteenth-century texts on line, for which scholars must be immensely grateful, and of references to material of whose existence they would not have previously been aware. The chance appearance on the internet of a photograph of a traveller's passing reference to Caius' annotations in a study of European relations with the Levant is only the most unlikely discovery. And one should not forget, the internet has made it possible to conduct a dialogue with distant colleagues that would have been impossible a generation ago. Despite their assistance, there will still be passages that remain obscure to readers unfamiliar with Caius' classical heritage and symbolism or whose significance in one way or another I have failed to recognise. But that is also one of the crucial features of this book, for in its language, its concepts and its expectations of its readership, it is in many ways typical of the work of European intellectuals in the middle years of the sixteenth century: they travelled, they corresponded, they wrote and they believed in a community of scholars united across the confessional divide.

The life of John Caius

A few street and house names apart, John Caius (1510–1573) is remembered today only in two institutions he served loyally and with distinction, although not always to the satisfaction of his fellow-members. In Cambridge, he used his considerable wealth to re-found his old college, Gonville Hall, in 1558, providing it with new buildings in the most up-to-date Italian style. The laconic epitaph on his splendid tomb in the College Chapel, '*Fui Caius*', 'I was Caius', expects the observer to know who he was, but the average tourist today is likely to be ignorant, as well as baffled by the local pronunciation of the usual name of Gonville and Caius College, Keys. The London College of Physicians, which he served as president nine times between 1555 and 1572, and whose history he wrote, displays in its Treasures Room several relics of his time, including his silver caduceus (a staff with two entwined snakes as its head). But the educational and medical ideals that he championed have long been superseded, and Caius himself soon after his death may have been reduced to a mere bit part in a Shakespearian comedy, *The Merry Wives of Windsor*.[3] In his life-time, however, he was one of the very few English scholars to enjoy a European reputation, and the last twenty-five years have seen a rehabilitation of much of his work, and particularly that on the manuscripts of Galen described in this autobibliography.[4]

John Caius was born and brought up in Norwich, a city for which he retained strong affection and where he made life-long contacts.[5] He dedicated one of his early works to an Alderman, Augustine Stiward, and planned, but never completed, a history of the city.[6] Two other students from Norwich School, Matthew Parker and William Framingham, were later to become his friends, and both enjoyed academic careers in Cambridge. Matthew Parker (1504–1575), six years Caius' senior, went on to become Master of Corpus Christi College, Cambridge, and subsequently archbishop of Canterbury.[7] He and Caius shared many interests, not least in history, both in Cambridge and in London, and Caius' writings on the history of Cambridge University drew on rare manuscripts in the archbishop's possession.[8] In the 1570s, when Caius was assailed for his opinions about religion and the proper governance of his college, and had his college rooms ransacked with the connivance, if not the participation, of the university authorities, he was still an honoured guest of Parker's in London.[9] William Framingham, by contrast with the celebrated archbishop, was a star that shone but briefly. Two years younger than Caius, he went up to Pembroke College, taking his BA in 1530/1, and immediately becoming a fellow of Queens'. His premature death in September 1537 at the age of twenty-five, was 'a greate losse of so notable a yonge man'.[10] As Caius wrote in English in 1552, in a passage summarised and turned into Latin in his *Autobibliography*, Framingham bequeathed to him all his writings, in Latin prose and verse. Their titles suggest that they were excellent examples of the new humanist literature, combining religious and moral exhortation in classical dress on the model of Erasmus. Caius, to whom Framingham had dedicated his book of epigrams, took on the task of preparing all this material for publication, writing commentaries to accompany the fair-copies provided for him by a pupil of Framingham, Nicholas Pergate. He had progressed so far with his task within a few months that he was able to send them off with a dedicatory letter to the Bishop of Norwich, Thomas Thirlby (1500–1570), who was a close friend of the author.[11] But Caius' move to Italy in 1539 proved disastrous for the project. The copy was passed by Thirlby to John Skippe (d. 1552), another Norfolk man and Bishop of Hereford, who in turn sent them on to Framingham's old tutor, Dr. Thixtill.[12] Thence they passed in succession to Sir Richard Moryson (1510–1556), the English ambassador at the imperial court, John Tailor (d. 1554), dean of Lincoln and a former fellow of Queens', and Sir Thomas Smith (1513–1577), the secretary of Henry VIII and another who overlapped with Framingham at Queens'.[13] But with Smith the trail ends, and on his return to England, Caius could find no trace of the manuscripts, although he continued searching at least until the 1570s. All he could hope for was that they would turn up in the end. The story of the missing manuscripts illustrates nicely two features of Caius' life: his loyalty towards his friends and his institutions, and the Cambridge, and in part East Anglian, network that linked him to church, state and the wider Europe.

He arrived at Gonville Hall on September 12, 1529, a little older than the majority of students. At this stage he probably thought of a theological career, for some of his early translations were of theological writings, and he knew Hebrew as well as Greek and Latin.[14] In a typically nostalgic digression in 1572 he contrasted contemporary students with his own generation, perpetually eager for the honour and glory of learning, proud to wear a cap and gown, properly dressed for lectures and chapel, and always giving way to their dons as they passed in the street. They keenly attended all their lectures in a spirit of cooperation and zeal for learning and dined together in a companionable spirit, taking a little wine only on high days and holidays. Removal from the university for moral turpitude was rare, while the highlight of their relaxation was participation in the Christmas plays.[15] This rosy picture of his life as a student and young don owes much to the troubles he encountered forty years later, but must also reflect his own success, first as a scholar of Gonville Hall, then heading the university list of graduations in early 1533, and finally as a fellow from December 1533 until 1545. But before his fellowship formally ended, he had left for Padua in March 1539 to pursue his studies in medicine.[16]

Although Caius nowhere explains his change of interest, Christopher Brooke makes the plausible suggestion that he was influenced by two senior members of the college, both royal physicians, Thomas Wendy (d. 1560) and William Butts (c. 1485–1565).[17] Wendy, the later dedicatee of one of Caius' editions of Galen, was often in Cambridge, since he lived in the nearby village of Haslingfield.[18] Butts, described by Caius as his patron in a reminiscence of their time together at Dover while he was on his way to Italy, acted as a major contact for Caians seeking positions at court and in London, where his evangelical sympathies appealed to Anne Boleyn and her circle.[19]

Medicine was not an obvious choice for a talented academic. Although it had long been taught in Cambridge, numbers of graduates were very few, fewer even than Oxford, and its teachers were undistinguished. It was to remedy this neglect that Thomas Linacre had established by his will a lectureship in medicine at St John's College in 1524, but it was not until 1540 that the Regius professorship of physic was founded.[20] Of the two known early Linacre lecturers, Christopher Jackson died suddenly in 1528, leaving behind little memory except a tombstone and his name in a few medical books.[21] His predecessor, George Day (c. 1502–1566), remained in Cambridge until 1543, and was praised by Caius for his medical learning and his wide-ranging activity as a teacher of rhetoric and other arts.[22] But both he and another early lecturer, William Bill (d. 1561), were more famous for divinity than for medicine, a subject that was then studied far more from books than in actual practice.

Linacre had founded his lectureships at Oxford and Cambridge with the aim of introducing into England the new humanist medicine as professed at

Italian universities such as Bologna, Ferrara and Padua. He himself was a graduate of Padua, which for half a century, following the ending of the Wars of the Roses, had attracted a steady stream of English students of medicine.[23] He had a European reputation as a translator from the Greek, especially of Galen, and he owned a major collection of Greek manuscripts. He was a distinguished grammarian, serving as a tutor as well as a physician to the family of Henry VIII. His example, as well as royal funds, encouraged others like John Clement and Edward Wotton, already well trained in Greek and Latin, to follow him to Padua and Italy.[24] Clement in particular, a medical graduate of Siena, had very close relations with Caius, although whether they began before or after Caius' Italian stay is not clear. Their careers and interests were very similar.[25] Clement had a remarkable fluency in Greek, having been a fellow at Corpus Christi College Oxford, and was one of editors of the first edition of the complete works of Galen in Greek, published by the Aldine Press in Venice in 1525–26. His library contained perhaps the best collection of Greek manuscripts in England, including the most important surviving manuscript of the Greek Anthology as well as numerous patristic writings, some of which he edited, to say nothing of medical texts.[26] Its dispersal in the sack of Malines in 1572, only a few weeks after his death, as well as his lengthy periods in exile, has hampered attempts to assess his importance within English and European humanism, but the quality of his scholarship is undeniable. He too enjoyed a successful medical career, becoming for a time a physician to Henry VIII, and in 1544 he was elected president of the College of Physicians. There were others in the London College, like Wotton, who had spent time in Padua, and whose example would have encouraged Caius to go abroad for his medical studies.

Italy had long been the Mecca for students from across the Alps.[27] The teachers of Bologna and Padua were rivals for pre-eminence, not least in medicine, and kept careful watch on developments in the other place. A decline in numbers of students at Padua in the early 1500s led to far-reaching Venetian reforms in 1517 which greatly strengthened the reputation of that university, not least by banning the granting of chairs to natives of the town.[28] Chief among the members of the medical faculty in the 1530s was the Veronese Giambattista Da Monte (1498–1551), the most authoritative Galenist of the day, famous not just for his knowledge of Galen but also for the way he put his master's precepts into practice.[29] His bedside teaching, already for some time a feature of Paduan training, was linked to his lectures on Galen, especially in their emphasis on proper method. Caius acknowledged his debt to Da Monte as his teacher, but his publication in 1544 of a version of Da Monte's lectures under his own name was apparently unauthorised and aroused the anger of others ostensibly more scrupulous.

Another northerner who came to Padua for his doctorate in medicine was Andreas Vesalius of Brussels (1514–1564), an ambitious young man with a remarkable talent for dissection (Figure 2). The day after obtaining his doctorate on December 5, 1537, he was appointed professor of anatomy and surgery and charged with conducting immediately the annual dissection on behalf of the medical faculty. Vesalius had no time to innovate, but students at his lectures the following year were faced with several novelties. Instead of the traditional system of a university anatomy, where one person read out passages from a set text, another cut up the corpse and a third explained what should be observed and put it into a context, Vesalius alone took charge, both dissecting and expounding what he was revealing. To accompany his

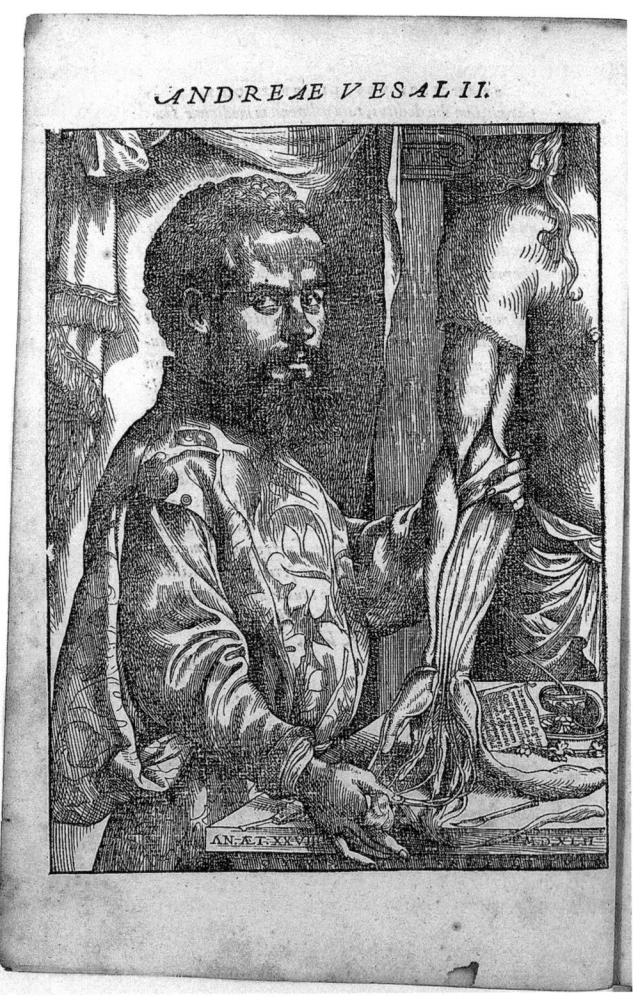

Figure 2 Andreas Vesalius (1514–1564). *Epistola rationem modumque propinandi radicis Chynae decocti*, Basle: J. Oporinus, 1546, frontispiece.

Copyright Wellcome Collection.

lectures, he further arranged for two different publications to be printed, both accessible to students in both language and price. One, paid for by the artist Jan van Calcar, was a series of six anatomical plates, the *Tabulae anatomicae sex*, illustrating the body and its parts and accompanied by brief notes. Although some schematic images of the body had already made their way into print, these were among the first, if not the first, to provide detailed illustrations to accompany a lecture course in anatomy.[30] He also provided a new textbook, his own revision of the *Principles of Anatomy according to Galen, Institutiones anatomicae secundum Galeni sententiam*, originally written by his Parisian teacher, Johann Guinter. Even more than the six plates, this verbal exposition shows a considerable movement away from the original doctrines of Galen.[31] Vesalius continued for a while to annotate his own copy in preparation for a revised edition, but by the time Caius came to know him, he had already changed his plan and had embarked instead upon the writing of his masterpiece, the *De humani corporis fabrica, The Fabric of the Human Body*, published by Oporinus at Basle in 1543.[32]

Caius and Vesalius were for a time close friends.[33] Caius, although he does not specifically say so, will have attended his anatomical dissections (something unknown in Britain at the time) and gained from them and from his discussions with Vesalius an enthusiasm for anatomy that he took back to London. The two men shared a house in Padua for several months, collaborating on a different anatomical project, a revision of the new humanist Latin versions of Galenic anatomy. The overall editor, Da Monte, had been engaged by the publishing firm of Giunta to superintend a massive new edition of the complete works of Galen in Latin translation. A collection of medieval translations of Galen had been published as long ago as 1490, but the publication of the Aldine edition of the original Greek in 1525–6, and still more, the outpouring from 1527 onwards of new translations based directly on the Greek rather than on Arabic or Hebrew intermediaries rendered these earlier complete editions obsolete. In what Caius termed 'honourable rivalry', below, p. 58, two Venetian publishers vied to be the first to produce a new collected edition. Not only would these editions bring together in one place translations of the Greek material made available for the first time in 1525–6, particularly Galen's commentaries and his writings on anatomy, but they would also improve on existing translations from the Greek by carefully comparing each word and phrase (the technical term is 'collating') against Greek manuscripts.[34]

It was a method that had been advocated with some success by Niccolò Leoniceno (1428–1524), the leader of the new medical humanists, at least from 1492, and was quickly adopted by other North Italian scholars with access to Greek manuscripts.[35] They had shown conclusively that many errors in the medieval translations were the result of a complex process of transmission, often involving at least three different languages, and that they could be frequently avoided by working directly from the Greek. But difficulties still remained. Editors and translators were (and are) fallible, and it was very quickly realised that the Aldine edition of the Greek was far from satisfactory as a basis from which to translate, for its printers were scarcely more accurate than the earlier medieval scribes. It had been put together in a great hurry, and the accident with the candle described by Caius, below, p. 70, was not the only source of confusion. Editing a text from manuscript for the first time is no easy task, and not all of the original group of editors were equally competent, but given the speed with which they worked, it is remarkable how much they achieved and how well they performed their task.

Nonetheless, improvements were there to be made, at first through a better understanding of Galen's Greek and conjectural emendation. One of the editors associated with the Aldine press in 1525–6, the German Georg Agricola (1494–1555), is said to have filled several books with conjectures, alas now lost.[36] His colleague in this enterprise, John Clement, scribbled many corrections in the margin of his copy of the edition, now in Leiden, many of which he sent on to Basle for use in the revised edition of the Greek that was published there in 1538.[37] Other editors, including Caius in some of his editions, attempted also to reconstruct the Greek by translating back from the medieval Latin versions, several of which, particularly those by Niccolò da Reggio (active from 1308–1346), had translated Galen's Greek faithfully word for word.[38] Although Caius had scrupulously recorded variant readings from Latin versions in his marginalia in his Eton Galen, he was also aware of the problems that they raised, devoting a long paragraph to warning against undue reliance on the Latin, something he thought was a common source of error.[39] But there was also the possibility of finding new texts and better and more accurate manuscripts that would permit a return to the exact words of the great Galen. It was not a foolish hope (although its limitations were not then fully realised), especially because the Aldine editors had relied on only a small number of Greek manuscripts from a relatively restricted area of Italy.

Second, the activities of collectors and the opening up of private libraries like that of the Medici in Florence or the Grimani collection at S. Antonio di Castello in Venice (below, pp. 78, 101) meant that more manuscripts were becoming available to those who made the effort to search for them. This was not easy, as Caius wishes his reader to understand. It demanded a substantial expenditure of time, as well as a network of contacts around Europe. Once located, a manuscript required careful and detailed collation, listing variant readings that might lead to an improved text of Galen. And, in turn, an improved text might lead to a better understanding of what he had recommended and to even better therapy. Not everyone had the skills, or the patience, to carry out this procedure, as Caius himself accepted. On the front sheet of the first volume of the Eton Galen, he wrote that restoring Galen required enormous effort, but one that helped both sides, for Galen had benefited Caius, and vice versa.[40]

It was a methodology vigorously followed by the two competing Italian groups, one led by Antonio Ricci and Vettore Trincavelli in Venice, the other by Agostino Gadaldino, the head of the Aldine press, and by Da Monte in Padua.[41]

Vesalius was commissioned by his Paduan colleague to revise the anatomical sections of Galen, a wise choice both because of his anatomical expertise and because he was an excellent classical scholar.[42] Gadaldino provided him with notes and some fragmentary manuscripts, which he collated at home with Caius.[43] If, according to Caius, Vesalius' translation was not as accurate as he would have wished, and the advantage gained from consulting these manuscripts negligible, this did not invalidate the methodology itself, which Caius followed studiously for the rest of his life, as we shall see. Not only did he find material that had been hidden for centuries, but he was able to produce a more accurate text and a better translation than any that had gone before.[44] His experience of the vagaries of medieval scribes led him to cast doubt on chapter headings in one text and on the order of books in another, while his reconstruction of a lost Hippocratic text from scattered indications, although flawed, is remarkable in its methodology.[45] Over the last thirty years Galenic scholars have begun to appreciate the value of his annotations in Eton and Cambridge for reconstructing the text of Galen and its *fortuna* in the Renaissance.

Vesalius left for Basle in 1542 to see the *Fabrica* through the press of Oporinus, but by then Caius had moved to share a house with a man from Como who took only bitter and acid drinks, a Milanese who drank only hot water and ate biscuit instead of bread, and another (if this is not Caius himself) who enjoyed only sweet drinks.[46] He took his doctorate in medicine on May 13, 1541, by which time he had already been appointed to lecture publicly on Aristotle in Greek, a very junior and poorly paid position, but one that provided him with an additional income to supplement his stipend as a Cambridge fellow, below, p. 66.[47] He was still lecturing in early 1543, when he had to compete for students with Realdo Colombo, Vesalius' assistant and temporary successor as professor of anatomy, who was teaching at the same time, below, p. 66. He says nothing of his other activities in Padua, except for his attempt to teach privately another Englishman Henry Knolles, and for his composition in 1542 of his *Method of Healing according to the Princes of Medicine, Galen of Pergamum and Giambattista Da Monte of Verona*.[48] This version of Da Monte's lectures, published at Basle in 1544, was strongly criticised by Johann Crato von Crafftheim (1519–85), another of Da Monte's students, who was himself later to publish a summary of the same lectures.[49] The several pages in his *Autobibliography* devoted by Caius to defending his publication are far from convincing.

His experience with Vesalius and Gadaldino seems to have strengthened his plan to edit many, if not all, of the writings of Galen, and to that end, as well as to meet other distinguished scholars, he embarked on a tour that took him as far South as Rome.[50] His *Autobibliography* provides a brief account of where he went and what he found that can be confirmed in part from the hundreds of annotations that he wrote in the margins of his copy of the 1538 edition of the complete works of Galen, now at in the library of Eton College, classmark Fc 2.6–8.[51] He mentions visiting Venice, Ferrara, Bologna, Pesaro, Urbino, Rome, Florence and Pisa, where he managed also to attend some lectures by the celebrated Galenist professor Matteo Corti, at the newly refounded university.[52] Some of the libraries whose holdings he examined had long been famous, such as that of S. Domenico at Bologna, others, like those at S. Domenico and SS Angeli in Ferrara, had only recently received major collections; still others, like the Marciana and the Grimani libraries in Venice, p. 78, had not previously been easily accessible. His status in the world of Italian scholarship also gained him entry to the private collections of its leading professors. His tour resembles that of another northern student in Padua, the Dutchman, Pieter van Foreest (1522–97), whose time there over-lapped with Caius' and who also claims to have attended some of Vesalius' dissections.[53] But neither man mentions the other, and although both were vigorous Galenists, Caius' interests in medical philology and in anatomy were rather different from the clinical concerns of Van Foreest, who later became the personal physician to William the Silent and the first professor of medicine at the new University of Leiden.

Caius had set himself a heavy task, not least because the five volumes of his Galen themselves weigh a total of 15 kg in their modern binding. Although at times he met with disappointment, he did succeed in discovering some works attributed to Galen in Greek that had not been known before, some of which he brought back and gave to his college.[54] Recent scholarship on Galen has enabled many of the manuscripts he mentions in this book to be identi-fied, and has also allowed an estimate of their value for the reconstruction of Galen's words.[55] He took notes on many manuscripts that were far superior to the text of either the Aldine or the Basle edition, but the most valuable entries may be those he took down from annotated copies owned by English scholars, most notably John Clement, which are now lost.[56] His final plea for scholars to do what he did and to improve the text of Galen has, in fact, become a reality only in the last century, and perhaps only in the last thirty years, when the significance of his Eton notes has been properly assessed.[57]

But it must also be admitted that the result of his labours was not as great as he had hoped. His improvements to the text of Galen, however philologi-cally satisfying and important for a more accurate translation, did not alter significantly the general thrust of Galen's medical ideas. They might change a word here and there, but in general the discrepancies between the Galenic texts themselves or, increasingly, between them and medical reality could not be resolved philologically. Even if many doctors continued to adhere to the Renaissance maxim of returning *ad fontes*, to the sources, and even if Galen's many treatises on therapeutics and pharmacology continued to be consulted for centuries to come, new syntheses, incorporating new discoveries or deal-ing with new diseases, to say nothing of Vesalian anatomy, came to supersede the words of the master. This was a slow process and one by no means as obvious to physicians in the 1560s and 1570s as it is today.

Caius' departure from Italy in 1544 marked the end of an era. As religious tensions mounted, the number of English students in Padua dropped consid-erably. Only those of Catholic sympathies now dared to study there. Some remained permanently in Italy, others, on their return to England, became vigorous proselytisers for the old religion.[58] It was not for a further forty years that significant numbers of English students began returning to Padua, lawyers first, medics five or six years later, and only then can one talk of a resumption of ties that had once been familiar.

It was on his way back to Cambridge that Caius may well have met personally, either in Zurich or in Basle, a man who was to have a profound influence on the rest of his life, Conrad Gessner (1516–65) [Figure 3].[59] Gessner was a polymathic physician, a prolific writer and a scholar with a Europe-wide reputation and contacts.[60] He edited and translated classical texts, including helping with the Basle 1562 edition of the Latin works of Galen, to which

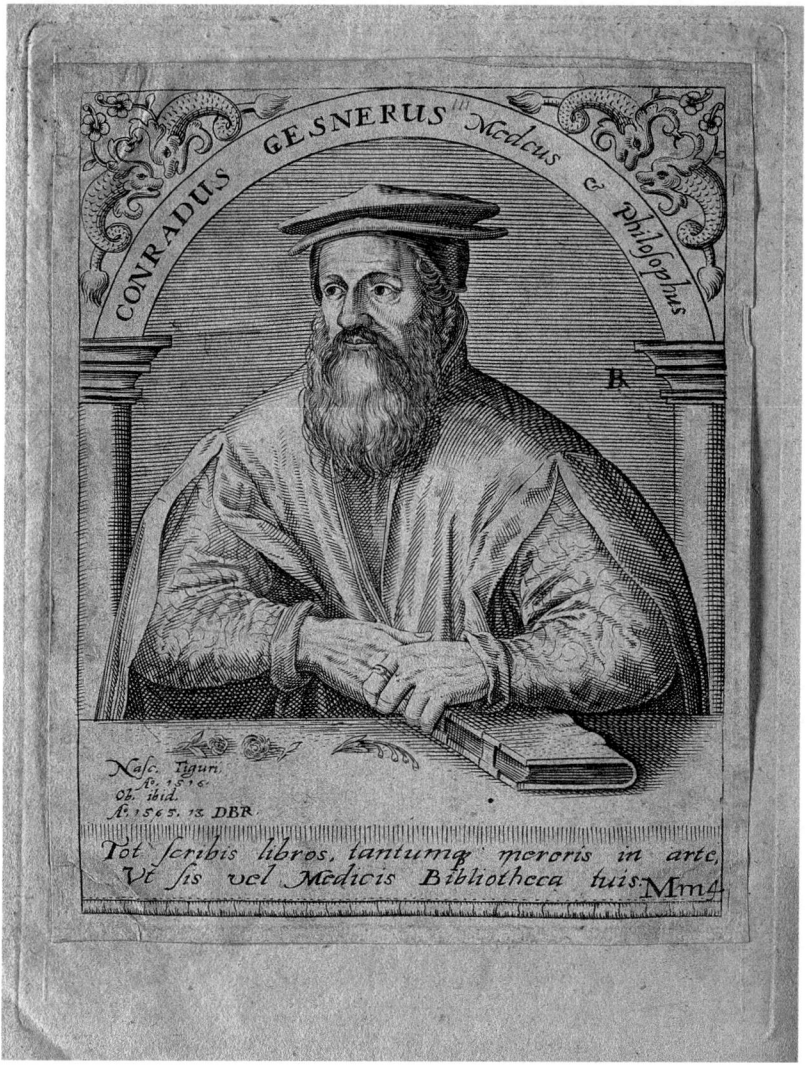

Figure 3 Conrad Gessner (1515–1565). Engraving by T. De Bry, 1650.

he contributed a major preface and comments on the authenticity of various treatises contained therein.[61] He was a bibliographer: his *Biblioteca universalis, A Universal Bibliography*, (1545) is possibly the first attempt to produce a catalogue of all known publications and had very soon to be extended by an appendix of new printings.[62] Above all, like many other physicians, he was a keen student of natural history, although in 1543 he had not yet begun to publish his *Historia animalium, An Enquiry into the Animal World*, a comprehensive account of all known animals, birds and fishes. Doctor, schoolmaster and author, he conducted, mainly from his home city of Zurich, a correspondence with scholars across Europe, seeking information on the latest discoveries of plants, animals, birds, fishes and other natural phenomena for inclusion in his publications. He shared many of his interests with Caius, and from the 1540s until Gessner's death, the two men exchanged books and passed on news to each other.[63] Caius sent him descriptions and drawings of rare animals and British dogs for inclusion in the revised version of Gessner's *Icones animalium (Images of Animals)*, and was acknowledged appropriately (Figure 4).[64] Even if they never did meet face to face, Gessner made a great impression on Caius at a human level. Gessner's death devastated him, and brought forth a remarkable lament for his lost friend, below, pp. 73–78.

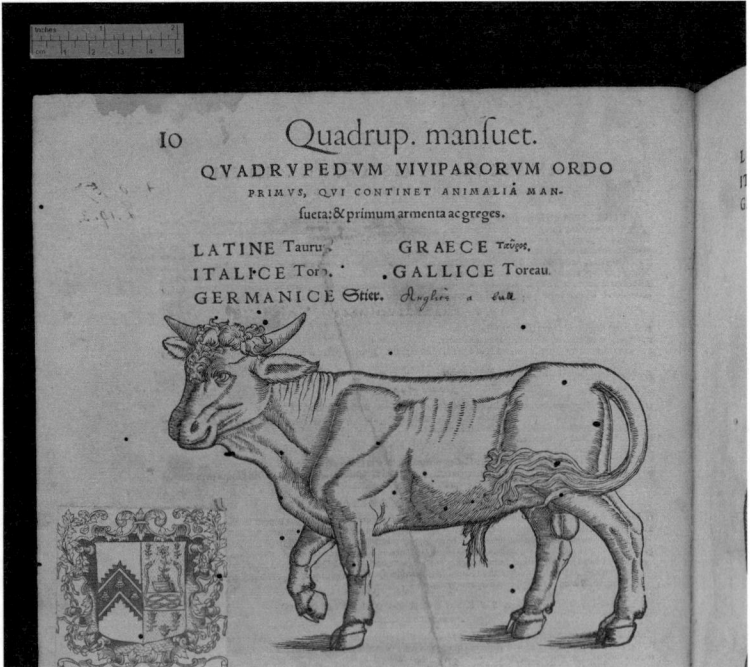

Figure 4 Conrad Gessner, *Icones animalium*, Zurich, 1560, Gonville and Caius College Library, L. 19.4, p. 10. Caius adds '*Anglice* a bull' to the original image in the book sent to him by Gessner.

The only letter surviving independently from what must have been a considerable correspondence, a letter of Gessner of August 29, 1561, to John Caius 'a most celebrated physician (*medico clarissimo*)' neatly encapsulates their relationship.[65] One of the longest letters in the published selection of Gessner's correspondence, in its present form it opens brusquely with a reference to a letter from William Turner (d. 1568), another British naturalist, and to Caius' intention to delay his book on British springs until he felt completely satisfied with it.[66] Gessner himself had written about such waters in Switzerland (and knew of other writers in other regions), and hoped to be able to mention Caius' work in a future publication. He himself had been away for a month in the mountains, taking the waters for health reasons, and at the same time examining their mineral properties. Had England, he wondered, any acidulous waters? He then moved on to the vexed question of the (non-)publication of John Claymond's commentary on the Roman Pliny's *Natural History*, about which Caius has much to say in his *Autobibliography*, below, p. 65. He could understand his friend's frustration at Oporinus' delay in printing this great work of scholarship: he was a good man and an excellent printer, but somewhat dilatory at times, not least because of his enormous output. Gessner offered his services in finding out what had happened and if necessary, in arranging for the transfer of the manuscript to another Basle printer, Froben. He was sympathetic, for he had recently had a bad experience himself with a printer from Strasbourg, who had failed to live up to his promises, and printed the medical writings of Valerius Cordus (1515–44) so badly that Gessner was ashamed to be associated with the book.[67] The rest of this wide-ranging letter is taken up with the identifications of various plants, fishes and animals made by Gessner, Caius and a variety of other scholars around Europe. As well as their publications Caius and Gessner exchanged specimens of leaves and twigs to back up their arguments; Gessner promised to send copies of the edition of Cordus and his own little tract on oxymel, which, along with some other recipes, he hoped would benefit his friend. Alas, Caius' new translations of works by Galen, which had been recently sent him, had arrived just too late to be included in the Froben edition of Galen that was already in press – only the index needed to be finished – but Gessner hoped to be allowed to retain a copy until the next edition was published.[68]

This letter reveals the close friendship between the two men, as well as the international network of scholarly correspondents of which they were a part.[69] Gessner sent letters to Italy almost every day, and he cited scholars and publications from France, Germany, Belgium and Italy, as well as Britain, who were engaged in the enterprise of finding new species and identifying correctly those mentioned in Greek and Latin texts from antiquity.[70] This interest in natural history united men of very different theological outlook, ranging from William Turner, Dean of Wells and John Parkhurst (1512–1575), the evangelical bishop of Norwich, both exiles on the continent under Mary Tudor, to George Bullock (1520/1–1572), Lady Margaret Professor and

Master of St John's College, Cambridge, who went into exile under Mary's sister Elizabeth.[71] Bullock, who brought letters from Caius while on his way to Italy, had enquired about a possible index for Gessner's *Partitiones theologicae (Theological Bibliography)*, and Gessner hoped that he would in turn be able to bring back to England news (and specimens) of some of Gessner's latest discoveries, although his optimism also shows how little he knew of the developing religious tensions within England in the 1560s.[72]

By then the four volumes of Gessner's great *Historia animalium* had set new standards in natural history. Caius had copies of all four volumes in his library, two with dedications to Caius as a 'distinguished doctor and philosopher in London' by Gessner himself, and he continued to correspond with new information until Gessner's death.[73] In turn, Gessner invoked Caius' aid in 1561 in resolving a tricky problem of protocol. The previous year Gessner had dedicated the second edition of his *Images of Animals* to Queen Elizabeth but without obtaining her permission.[74] He had come to hear that she was displeased at this, perhaps because the first edition of 1553 had been dedicated to Thomas and John, the brothers of Henry Grey, Duke of Suffolk (1517–1554), 'the sun among lesser constellations', all Protestant sympathizers with close links to the evangelicals in Zurich. Henry Grey himself was married to a niece of Henry VIII, and the father of Jane and Catherine Grey, 'distinguished for their attainments in Latin and Greek as well as for their modesty'. Their royal connections and their piety would have made the family appropriate recipients of Gessner's florid dedication.[75] But within months all had changed. Lady Jane Grey (1537–1554) was made queen on the death of Edward VI, and although Henry Grey himself was not implicated in the plot, he was very soon likewise executed on the orders of Queen Mary for opposing her marriage to Philip of Spain. Choosing Elizabeth as a replacement for members of such a family, and without her permission, was at best tactless and showed, at the very least, ignorance of the religious and political situation in England. Gessner was forced to write apologetically to William Cecil, saying that he had explained everything very fully in a letter to Caius, whom he wished Cecil to use as an intermediary when he replied, if, indeed, he ever chose to broach the subject with the queen.[76] Since he was a poor man with many relatives to support, Gessner pleaded that he might be paid at least the four crowns that it had cost him to send the book. Cecil did his best and was successful, for a few weeks later Gessner received the not inconsiderable sum of six pounds, presumably as recompense for his work.[77]

Caius retained his links with Basle long after he had returned to England. As well as the edition of some Geek texts of Galen published by Froben and Episcopius (Caius 1544b) and his own *Method of Healing* (Caius 1544a), he issued further editions and translations of Galen with Froben in 1549 and with Oporinus in 1557, and planned to send others to Froben.[78] As we have seen, he also tried without success to have John Claymond's commentary on Pliny printed by Oporinus, and his own further selection of Galenic texts suffered a similar fate (below, p. 65).

But detailed information on where he went and what he did after his departure from Basle in 1544 is sparse. He mentions three distinguished German scholars, Philip Melanchthon (1497–1560), Joachim Camerarius the Elder (1500–1574) and Sebastian Münster (1488–1552), for their retention of the old, pre-Erasmian pronunciation of Greek, claiming to have been on friendly terms with them all. The Hebraist and cosmographer Münster he may well have met in Basle, where he taught at the university, but when, or indeed if, he met the two others is problematical. Neither lived in a town on an obvious direct route to Italy, although Camerarius was still teaching in 1539 at Tübingen on the Neckar, which would have involved a detour of only a few days. But in 1541 he moved to the distant Leipzig, relatively close to the Wittenberg of Melanchthon, and a visit to him after that date would have taken a considerable time. Given the uncertainty over the date of Caius' arrival in Padua, a visit to Wittenberg to visit Melanchthon on his way out cannot be excluded entirely, although this would have involved a much longer detour, and Raven's suggestion of one in 1543 is also questionable.[79] But Caius' description of their friendship is ambiguous, and his knowledge of their pronunciation could easily have been gained indirectly from others who knew the two men personally or, since he calls them friends, through correspondence. Their names are introduced not just to support his theories, but also to buttress his credentials as a scholar, and in the wider context, as a friend of three of the leading European Protestant scholars.

But both here and elsewhere in his writings Caius gives more specific information on his activities, even if they cannot always be dated precisely. He explicitly refers to hearing some of the professors at Louvain, p. 79, but without saying whether this was on his way to Italy or, more likely, on his return journey. He almost certainly returned briefly to Cambridge to see out the end of his fellowship in September 1545, but for the next decade and more, London was the centre of his activities. In 1547, he was elected a fellow of the London College of Physicians, and encouraged by Henry VIII, also began about this time a series of lectures to the Barber Surgeons on the theory and practice of anatomy. In 1550 he set up house within the precincts of St Bartholomew's hospital, although he does not appear to have held any hospital position.[80] In his writings he mentions visits to Kenilworth, Warwick, Kings Lynn, Selsey, Boston and Orford, but his account of the arrival of the English Sweat in Shrewsbury in 1551 need not derive from any experience there.[81] These and a few references to other patients in Essex and Kent do not suggest that he spent any length of time in any one place in the provinces, and it is probably best to assume that he spent most of his time in London.[82] He knew various members of the court, not least the Cecil and the Bacon families, but there is no secure evidence that he was ever officially employed as a royal physician.[83] Practice among the richer inhabitants of the capital would account for his acquisition of substantial wealth both in this poorly documented period and later.

Much of his time in the 1550s was spent on the affairs of the College of Physicians of London, as an elect, a councillor, censor and in 1555 president for the first time. The college had been founded in 1518 after a petition by Thomas Linacre and other royal physicians to Henry VIII.[84] An attempt a century earlier to create a similar institution to oversee medical practice had lasted only briefly, and there was no organisation for the physicians of London comparable to the Guild of Barbers and the Fellowship of Surgeons. To Linacre and his friends, many of whom had studied on the Continent, where such colleges had long been familiar, such an omission was a reproach to a modern monarchy and a danger to a city whose increasing size and wealth were attracting ever more practitioners of different skills and competences.[85] Their aim was two-fold: to set up an organisation that, as in Italy, regulated all medical practice in the city and that would impose proper standards of learning, by which they meant the new humanist medicine, on all those concerned with healing. They had wider ambitions, to extend their writ beyond the limits of the city to all England, but even their immediate plans faced difficulties that would continue for centuries.

The first was simply numerical. The number of fellows was always small (in 1518 there were twelve, and rarely more than twenty until the end of the century), and they were faced with a population rapidly growing to become the largest in Europe. Nor could the college expect a substantial flow of qualified entrants, for London, unlike Padua, had no local university whose graduates and professors could easily move into the college, and Oxford and Cambridge together produced only a handful of MDs in a decade. The two universities, miles from London, were as jealous of their privileges as the college was eager to impose its own, higher, standards on their members. Its criteria for membership included, at least from the 1540s, a stiff examination in the works of Hippocrates and Galen, something way beyond the capabilities of most of those who offered healing in the city and often, at least initially, of those who were later to become members.

But the major problem faced by the college was one of authority: how to enforce the powers that had been given them in 1518 and later. No matter how often the college might point to royal insistence on their rights to dictate how 'physic' should be practised or to examine all aspects of medicine, from inspecting pharmacists' shops (a standard element in the role of a continental college) to establishing a curriculum, others raised objections or disregarded the college entirely. Its members were a small elite, bound together by education and their work in city and court, and although having many powerful supporters among their patients, faced opposition from others who thought their own privileges infringed – the universities, the city of London, parliament, city guilds and even the bishop of London, who had also enjoyed rights of supervision of medical practice in and around London. All these were in a strong position to oppose the college's ambitions, unlike the man in the street, who might never have heard of the college and who certainly could not afford its members' fees to treat family illnesses. The early history of the college is filled with such challenges, few of which it successfully repelled, save in one period, that described by its historian as that of 'John Caius and resolute action'.[86]

Caius became president for the first time in 1555. He quickly set to work organising the college's financial and secretarial accounts, as well as making changes to the statutes over a period of some years. He pursued with vigour those who disobeyed the college's rules.[87] In 1556, the college obtained a letter from the commissioners appointed by Cardinal Pole to review the universities, warning Oxford not to admit anyone to a medical degree without an appropriate course of study. An Oxford request to examine and punish unqualified practitioners there and for seven miles around seems also to have been rejected. Caius also issued a general warning over what he regarded as the pretensions of the apothecaries, whose subordination to the Physicians was confirmed in 1558 in a letter to the apothecaries from Queen Elizabeth herself. The years immediately before 1560 mark the high watermark of the college's successes in enforcing their authority, largely because it could obtain backing from both Mary and Elizabeth and from their ministers: many fellows, for example, will have known Cardinal Pole well during time spent in Padua. But Caius himself was increasingly occupied in another great project, and his energy and enthusiasm were diverted elsewhere, to the refounding of his old Cambridge college.

There is no need here to recount in detail the processes whereby in 1557 Caius obtained a charter for the refounding of Gonville Hall, his subsequent election as Master in 1559, and his substantial rebuilding of the college between 1563 and 1569.[88] All this was made possible by the substantial wealth that he had amassed from his activities as a physician based in London, much of which he had invested in property that he made over to the college. His energy was formidable, and once embarked upon a project, he strove vigorously to complete it, even if his methods aroused opposition. A capable administrator himself, he had little patience with what he saw as incompetent administration in others. On becoming Master, he expressed his horror at finding everything neglected and close to bankruptcy. Few knew anything about college business or property; legal deeds had been lost or scattered about; and chapel utensils had been removed for private use.[89] In his battle to restore (and conserve) order, history played a part. As with the London College, Caius himself took on the task of writing up the history of the college, not only to serve as an incentive to future generations but more immediately to record these momentous changes.[90] He also insisted that the annual record be continued by a fellow of the college. History mattered to Caius, particularly in defending causes he held dear. His restoration of the tomb of Linacre in St Paul's Cathedral is on a par with his much-derided attempt to prove the greater antiquity of Cambridge University against the claims of an Oxonian Caius, a wondrous mixture of fact and imagination, not all of which was his own invention.[91] His *History of Cambridge University* is less fanciful, and its detailed description of both town and gown a remarkable and unusual achievement.[92] Both books depended on a substantial engagement with earlier historians and with archives in both university and college collections, a passion he shared with Archbishop Parker and others in his London circle. But the great learning and ingenuity that his writings display are not always accompanied by an equivalent critical sense or a passion for accuracy; advocacy at times takes precedence.[93] Like his autobibliography, his historical works have an overtly exhortatory purpose beyond the simple desire to shape future interpretation of events as he would have wished.[94] History, in the view of Caius and that of most of his contemporaries, serves to remind the present of the achievements of the past that others would do well to emulate.

Caius was also a moderniser, not least in the building of the new college courts and gates; their architecture and decoration reflected the latest Italian styles, while the opening up of one court on one side let in fresh air that, according to recent theory, would reduce infection. A draft in English talks of restricting fellowships and scholarships to those not particularly well off, and, as well as insisting on the study of Greek up to the degree of MA, demands that its students should aim for 'summe necessarie office in the Common wealth', in medicine, law or theology.[95] He insisted on high standards for his future physicians. In 1564, he obtained permission for the college to acquire two bodies a year so that it could have two annual dissections, in addition to any provided by the university, something unheard of elsewhere.[96]

But he also looked backwards to an almost idealised time in his youth. His first visit to Cambridge in 1558 after his long absence in London was a disappointment; he knew no-one, and no-one knew him, and everything from student behaviour to the pronunciation of Greek had changed for the worse.[97] His Statutes are an attempt to restore this lost age, giving the Master power to dismiss 'his' Fellows and punishing severely with expulsion students (and perhaps even Fellows) who might presume to enter the college by any route save the gates. The list of conditions that should disqualify anyone from membership, such as blindness or mutilation, is traditional, save for the addition of '*Wallicum*', an ambiguous spelling that has led to considerable debate as to whether Caius disliked Welshmen or syphilitics.[98] Fussy and verbose these regulations might seem today, but that is typical of statutes, and they do attempt to put into effect a noble vision of what an education might be. Caius himself seems to have been scrupulous in his attention to detail and precise in his administration, and expected others to be the same.[99]

Reality, and human nature, got in the way. Caius was dissatisfied with much he saw around him, from the practice of coddling children with hot buttered toast and the extravagant fashions of undergraduates to the unwillingness of some junior Fellows to behave as he thought fit.[100] The London College at this period had also become involved in several unsuccessful attempts to punish practitioners supported by great Protestant magnates, and its willingness to accept Paduan graduates of doubtful Elizabethan orthodoxy only exacerbated the hostility of the new regime.[101] Never a man to shrink from confrontation, he began his treatise on pronunciation with two pages in favour of a conservative scepticism about all kinds of novelty: 'wiser men prefer old wine to new'.[102] By the time he came to complete his autobibliography in 1570, he was beginning to feel his years, 'I am senior but not senile' (he was 60 or so), but he was far from finished.[103] He had only recently completed the rebuilding of his college, and had plans for the future, or at least for the publication of books he now considered 'ripe' and for resuming his work on Norwich and on many Galenic texts.

He could also look back with satisfaction on what he had achieved. A religious conservative, he had nonetheless survived the difficult years of the 1560s, which saw other college heads deposed and driven into exile.[104] He had effectively finished his rebuilding and reorganisation of his college, and it was only a few years since he had played a leading role in welcoming the queen herself on an official visit to Cambridge.[105] He could lay claim to friendships across the religious spectrum, from Melanchthon, Camerarius and Münster on the Continent, p. 79, to the Clement family, devoted keepers of the legacy of Thomas More, and to English Protestant luminaries like William Cecil and Archbishop Parker.[106] His account of a dinner with Parker and Bishop Guest of Rochester, below, p. 55, shows that he was still held in high regard by those prelates at the end of his life, and he retained close links with the London historians and antiquaries.[107] Surrounded by like-minded friends in his Cambridge College, apparently secure in the protection of some of the highest in the land, unwilling to follow Clement and other acquaintances into exile, and perhaps also misjudging the speed with which academic differences could be turned into much more dangerous divergences in theology and politics, he could remain optimistic and still look to a productive old age.[108]

But his enemies were gathering. In 1572 his religious views led to a letter of complaint to Edwin Sandys, the bishop of London, who wrote 'very earnestly' to the vice-chancellor.[109] His response was to organise a raid on Caius' rooms, which ended with three hours of looting, burning what could be burnt and smashing what could not. Whether this included his books on theology and history is not clear, but they do not appear in the posthumous inventory of his books in London. Caius retreated to London, where he became so ill that he was unable to visit his friend the archbishop. Some even supposed that he had been banned from the archbishop's house.[110] His final visit to his college was by litter on June 23, 1573. Conscious of his impending death, he resigned his mastership four days later, spending the next few days planning for his funeral and for his tomb before returning to London, where he died at home on July 29. His will made over almost all his estate to the college, enjoining them to attend always to the repair of Linacre's tomb in St Paul's cathedral (later destroyed in the Great Fire of London in 1666) and to 'emplloye a lustie and helthie honeste trewe and unmaried man' of forty or over to sweep the paths and gutters within and without the college, to open and shut the gates and to light the lanterns in winter. He gave his books to the college (although not all those in his inventory are now be found there), and his own manuscripts to Archbishop Parker, some of which he saw through to publication. His tomb in the college chapel bears on its entablature the words: *vivit post funera virtus*, 'virtue lives on after death', words that he had applied to his greatest friend, Conrad Gessner, p. 76 below, and had had inscribed on the tomb of Thomas Linacre. It is a fitting conjunction.[111]

The scholar and his books

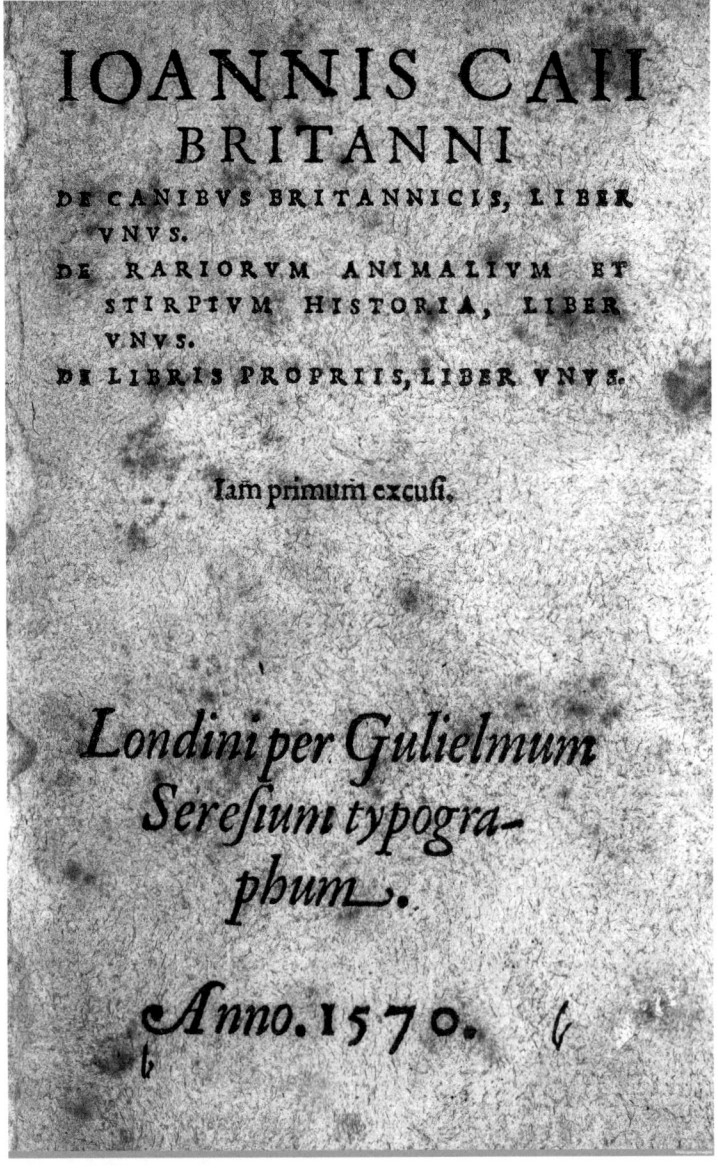

Figure 5 Caius, *De libris propriis*, 1570. Title page.

At first sight, Caius' autobibliography, *De libris propriis*, literally *On my own Books*, is a simple book, an account of his own writings. The reader is told a good deal about the contents of his many works, and often the circumstances under which they were written. The incidents in his life he chooses to include relate closely to them. Thus, there is relatively little mention of his activities as a practitioner, a leading member of College of Physicians or the re-founder and subsequently Master of Gonville and Caius College. But a careful reading reveals contradictions and complexities beginning with the very title, which differs in Latin from that given inside the book, see below, p. 84, note 1. Some of Caius' works which were still unpublished at the time of writing later appeared in print, although the extent to which they were revised after 1570 is far from clear; others, like the *History of Norwich*, if they were ever completed, are now lost.[112] There are also passages that cannot easily be characterised as bibliography, but are more in the nature of personal reactions, for example to the death of Gessner or the new pronunciation of Greek.

There are also indications that the book went through several stages before being printed in 1570. Even if one chooses not to believe Caius' statement, pp. 79–80, that it was begun during his Italian tour, at which point he had published nothing, he had certainly prepared a short version for Gessner in the early 1550s, which he later revised. His uncertainty over the manuscripts he left with Johann Oporinus also implies a composition at different dates. The abrupt and asyndetic nature of his comments on others' views on the pronunciation of Greek and Latin, p. 79, very different from his otherwise elegant periodic style, might also indicate that he had not yet fully revised his manuscript, although other explanations are possible.

Written in the form of a letter to the importunate Thomas Hatcher, his *Autobibliography, De libris propriis*, was intended for a much wider audience, one of fellow scholars and doctors, as the final appeal emphasises. By choosing Latin, the universal language of learned Europe, Caius made it clear that he was aiming at a readership in England and beyond that knew him as one of the most eminent Galenists and naturalists of his day.[113] They may not have all appreciated the names of English ambassadors and politicians mentioned as friends or dedicatees, but everyone with any pretensions to culture knew those of Sebastian Münster, Joachim Camerarius and Philip Melanchthon, and understood what it meant to be on terms of friendship with them.[114] The long list of his books establishes Caius as a prolific scholar, while the names of those with whom he enjoyed cordial relations further indicates that his eminence was acknowledged by intellectuals all over Europe.

To define oneself by one's books was not new. The most famous of all renaissance scholars, Desiderius Erasmus (1466? –1536), had produced a catalogue of his own writings in 1523 which went through several revisions before it achieved its final form in the prefatory matter to the collected edition of his works published by Froben in 1540. Like Caius, Erasmus interspersed the details of his books with some personal data and reflections.[115] Conrad Gessner had also published a similar, if more succinct, list under his own name in the various editions of his *Bibliotheca universalis* and, separately, in a letter that he wrote to William Turner in 1562.[116] The latter was subsequently reused by Josias Simler as an appendix to his biography of Gessner, published in 1566.[117] Given his admiration for both authors, it is probable that Caius knew some or all of these books, but none features in the inventory of his library in London, although, if Philip Grierson's suggestion is right, Caius did own a copy of Simler and Lycosthenes' *Epitome* of the *Bibliotheca*.[118] But neither Erasmus nor Gessner displays the range of personal detail included by Caius, who was also a far less prolific writer.

For that combination Caius had a model familiar to him for many years, Galen's treatise of the same title that he had himself edited and translated in 1556. Written by Galen (c. 129–c. 216) towards the end of his life, it prefaced a detailed account of his writings with a description of his early career that, together with information provided in the much earlier treatise, *Prognosis*, has continued to provide the basis for all subsequent biographies of Galen. Ostensibly written to settle a dispute over which of the many treatises circulating under his name was genuine or misattributed, it reveals much about Galen's background and education. It was not strictly autobiographical – there would have been much more information in a work, now lost, entitled *Slander*, 'where there is also something about my life', but, like *My own Opinions*, it was intended to establish Galen's true position in the face of the misrepresentations and misunderstandings of others.[119] Like so much else in Galen, it preached the gospel of Galen, setting out how just he wished to be perceived by others, not only through an emphasis on certain events and individuals, but more subtly, through its silences and omissions.

While one can be certain that Caius knew this tract of Galen extremely well, it is not at all clear that he was acquainted with another medical autobiography that also took Galen as its model. Girolamo Cardano (1501–1576) had printed his own list of writings for the first time in 1539, and published a much larger version in 1544, under the title *De libris propriis*. This in turn appeared in ever more revised versions, in 1557 and 1562, and culminated in the far less bibliographical *De propria vita*.[120] Although this is the version of his life that is most celebrated today, it is worth remembering that it was not published in Cardano's lifetime, and indeed not until 1643. Although it appealed to the example of Galen and Erasmus, it became over time a very sophisticated and far more autobiographical account than theirs, or than Caius' for that matter.[121] It had an overtly polemical purpose, founded on the need to establish Cardano's credentials as one who preached a reformed and extended humoral medicine, and, as time went on, the bibliographical element in it diminished. Whether Caius had read any of it is uncertain, for Cardano was a controversial figure in academic circles. But, as a resident in London in 1552 with connections to the court, Caius can hardly have failed to have heard of Cardano's controversial visit to London ostensibly to treat Edward VI for chest problems.

Cardano had been introduced to the young king when on his way to Scotland in summer 1552 to attend John Hamilton, the archbishop of St Andrews, where, some weeks later, he received an invitation to return to examine the sickly monarch.[122] In London, he lodged with Sir John Cheke, the chamberlain and tutor to the young king and an acquaintance of Caius, where he quickly learned that he had been invited not only as a physician but by some court politicians also as a noted astrologer who would forecast the death of the sovereign. In a later justification of his conduct, he says that the stars foretold that the weakling king had only a few more months to live, but in his formal response he prudently chose to predict that this 'second Solomon' would not die until he reached the age of 56.[123] He left soon after via the Netherlands, having learned from Cheke that conditions in France made it dangerous for him to take the shorter way home with so many servants and so much cash. If Caius knew of this tactful prediction, and its swift failure, it would only have encouraged him to think of Cardano as a charlatan, and certainly not as a model to be followed.

That Galen's autobibliography was the major influence on Caius' own work is obvious from the many verbal reminiscences that can be found within it. The assertion at the beginning of the book that Caius had been reluctant to publish, and then agreed only in response to the importunings of a friend, recalls many such prefaces by Galen, while Thomas Maro's long attendance at Caius' anatomical lectures corresponds to Galen's comments on the ex-consul Flavius Boethus, the recipient of *Anatomical Procedures* and a spectator at many of Galen's Roman demonstrations.[124] But there are two major differences. The first is structural: Caius, as he himself admits, often digresses, and the work contains three long sections that break up the flow of the narrative: his defence against accusations of plagiarism, his explanation of his theory of a lost Hippocratic work on anatomy, and the long lament for Conrad Gessner. All these will be discussed in turn later and their role in establishing Caius' *persona* further examined.

The meditation on Gessner, with its tropes about the immutability of fate, pp. 73–78, is an example of a second difference from the Galenic model. As far as we know, Galen wrote *My own Books* with little or no recourse to his other writings. He may have been able to use a list of his own works, whether compiled by himself or by a servant, but none of the incidents described in that book was copied directly from an earlier presentation. Although Galen is never reluctant to reveal incidents from his own life, and felt passionately about presenting an account of his life and ideas that corresponded to what he himself had experienced and believed to avoid misrepresentations and misunderstandings by others, *My own Books* does not depend on what he had said or written earlier. His self-fashionings, as Raiola has shown, are tailored to the individual recipient at a particular time.[125] By contrast, despite Caius' protestation that he only decided to write when badgered into it by Thomas Hatcher, he incorporated into it much that he had written earlier both in Latin and in English. His repetitions are at times so exact that they rule out an explanation in terms of a similar theme or association of words (although there are examples of both), but must have been copied either from Caius' original manuscripts or, more likely, from earlier printings, for such self-references are easier to find on the shelves in a printed book than in a hand-written codex. They serve as a warning against taking this *Autobibliography* as a simple composition created at a single moment in time.

Whether the long account of Caius' edition of the writings of William Framingham, pp. 54–55, should be labelled a digression is a matter of individual judgment. What is clear is that, while it here opens appropriately a list of Caius' publications, it is irrelevant to the context in which it first appeared, the English version of his book on the sweating sickness. Neither Caius' unsuccessful attempts to publish his friend's works nor their contents fit a work in English on a medical topic aimed at a wider public, not all of whom could read Latin, let alone appreciate Framingham's expertise as a Latin versifier.[126] Given Caius' tendency to wander off the subject, one need not assume that he had already composed a draft of this Latin text (or of at least parts of it) as early as 1552, but the closeness of the two redactions indicates that, at the very least, Caius in his final version took over much of his earlier information, and may have translated the English into Latin, with suitable modifications. He added a mention of his own juvenile translation of a work ascribed to Nicephorus Callistus Xanthopoulus, but removed some references to local individuals, like Alderman Stiward of Norwich, inappropriate in a work intended for a wider European readership.

Placed at the very beginning of his book, the list of juvenilia stresses an aspect of Caius' behaviour that recurs throughout the work; his loyal friendship. It had been, and at the time of writing still was, his intention to bring together in a publication the scattered writings of his friend and schoolmate, rather as Thomas Hatcher himself had published the *Lucubrations* of Walter Haddon.[127] It was a mark of his loyalty to his friend, and to his native Norwich, and his failure to achieve his aim was due to his own kindness and generosity in allowing a draft to be circulated among his own friends and those who had known Framingham, above p. 7. The story of his attempts to publish Claymond's commentaries on Pliny can also be read in this light, p. 65. Similarly, the names included in this treatise form a list of the good and great in England and in the wider scholarly world, all of them either specifically or by implication introduced as his friends. Caius' description of his life with Vesalius in Padua, p. 58, suggests an intimacy with the famous anatomist that contrasts with his (later) vigorous criticism of the Fleming in the margins of his editions of Galen, and, still more, with his single direct reference to another distinguished anatomist, Realdo Colombo, as his competitor for a student audience.[128] Caius singles out two errors of Vesalius that he had already acknowledged in the 1555 second edition of the *Fabrica*, but in rejecting others' discoveries as either wrong, trivial or irrelevant to medical practice, he chooses examples where Vesalius' views, even if not identical with his own, were denied by Colombo in his treatise on anatomy.

Nowhere is the theme of friendship more apparent than in the long lament for Conrad Gessner, a digression that occupies seven pages in the original. Caius had lost a soul-mate, whose interests coincided considerably with his own. Although they can only have met personally for a few weeks at most, if at all, during Caius' return from Italy, their epistolary friendship continued for nigh on twenty years. It was a friendship of equals, and the surviving, gossipy letter of Gessner to Caius is ample testimony to their mutual admiration.[129] Gessner's death was a severe blow for Caius, who respected his friend's scholarship as well as a morality that transcended any sectarian divisions. His moral virtues were expressed in his scholarship. Not only was Gessner a prolific writer on theological and ethical topics, but his preface to the 1561/2 Froben edition of Galen contained a long, and to a modern investigator unsuccessful, attempt to hold up Galen as a model of the Christian virtues.[130] Yet those who have commented on Caius' remarkable meditation on his friend's death have failed to notice one striking feature: much of what he wrote in 1570 is not original, but taken almost verbatim from his 1556 Latin account of the English Sweat, where his lament for the human condition in general fits the context of an epidemic far better than the death of an individual, below, pp. 73–78. Verbal changes are few, and, as Caius himself appears to realise towards the end of the passage, the ancient Greek advice that life is so distressing that it is better not to be born, or at least to die quickly, is hardly suitable for a Christian who had lived to almost fifty. The borrowing is patent.

This lament, however, also offers a clue to how Caius hoped this treatise would be received. It is not an autobiography as such, for far too much is omitted or left ambiguous. Indeed, some of his other treatises reveal far more about himself and his attitudes to the world around him. But it is also more than a simple account of his own writings, being interspersed with what might seem to modern eyes rambling digressions and an excess of examples. But in the context of the renaissance world of learning, these discrepancies are less striking, and indeed contribute to an overarching argument. This book is a manifesto, setting out the reasons for Caius' success as a European scholar.

His scholarship is expressed not only in the hard labour of collation, edition and translation of ancient Greek and Latin texts, and in the painstaking, and occasionally unfruitful, search for copies of Galen and Celsus in Italy and elsewhere. There were also other features that learned contemporaries would have noted. The two long sections recalling his relationships with Framingham and Gessner attest the role of friendship in the interchange of scholars. In the first Caius performs a service for his dead friend, in the latter he recalls Gessner's to him. Two other sections show his expertise in anatomy and in philology, areas in which all true scholars could be expected to show an interest. Others show both his detailed knowledge of individuals and incidents from the classical world as well as his familiarity with some unusual authors.

The piling-up of examples from medicine and literature (not all of which may have been derived directly from his own reading of ancient sources) confirms his right to a European reputation. He is a master of the Latin periodic style, with long and complex Ciceronian sentences. He employs different stylistic levels, and it is unclear whether the long sentence, entirely in asyndeton, on the failings of his opponents to speak correct Greek and Latin, is a sign of incompleteness or a demonstration of his mastery of a different style.[131] His lament for Gessner, in part derived from a preface he had directed to a famous patron of humanists, Antoine Perrenot, the future Cardinal Granvelle (1517–1586), neatly links together quotations and allusions in treating a standard theme in humanist rhetoric. If linguistically he is not as innovative as an Erasmus or even Johann Guinter of Andernach, he uses a rich vocabulary effectively and generally clearly.[132] In a world that valued Latin as a social as well as an intellectual marker, Caius' book demonstrates that he is one of the elite. Theologians aside, few Englishmen of his day could claim such a wide European recognition, or write Latin so well.[133]

John Caius and Renaissance Galenism

Medicine came relatively late to the medieval universities and was always a minority subject compared with law, arts and, in Northern Europe, theology. Numbers of students were always small, except at Bologna, Paris and Padua, for the course was long and expensive, although the rewards in the end might be high. By 1270 there had developed a syllabus that remained relatively stable across Western Europe until the sixteenth century. It was based on texts by classical Greek authors, especially Galen and, to a lesser extent, the Hippocratic Corpus, as systematised and interpreted by writers in Arabic such as Avicenna and Haly Abbas, all translated and circulating in Latin. It emphasised the over-arching theory behind all medical practice, the celebrated theory of the four humours, blood, phlegm, bile and black bile, providing a complex account of illness as deriving from some imbalance between these humours. The aspiring physician was instructed in diagnosis and, particularly, prognosis, as well as in a range of therapies, but his knowledge was gained largely from reading and from lectures, often in the form of a commentary on a set text, and his engagement with patients during his training was on the whole brief. Surgery and manipulation were left to the 'mechanics', surgeons and barber-surgeons, who were allegedly less concerned with the overall health of the patient, which, so it was believed, was best judged by observation of a wide range of factors allied to careful reasoning. By understanding the constitution of the patient, in health as well as in sickness, the wise physician could prevent much illness and prescribe appropriate treatment by diet and drugs when it did occur. It was an intellectual system that could point to hundreds of years of apparent success, as well as explaining bodily changes that were obvious even to the unlearned.

It also demanded a rigour and sophistication comparable to that in law and philosophy, both equally dependent on a high level of theory and an expertise in the interpretation of texts.[134]

But although stable, it was not immutable. An annual dissection of a human corpse was introduced at the university of Bologna around 1317, to be followed soon after in Padua, but this innovation spread at first only slowly and sporadically. The most erudite professors in Italy and France also took advantage of the many short Galenic texts translated from Greek into Latin at Naples in the first four decades of the fourteenth century by Niccolò da Reggio, and their successors in the next century produced large series of *consilia*, exemplary case-histories and prescriptions, that were copied widely.[135] This was a Latin medicine (vernacular translations were few, and medical books in languages other than Latin were confined almost entirely to self-help manuals or to surgery) discussed and developed by writers in Latin who had little direct access to any originals whether in Greek, Arabic or Hebrew.

The arrival of Greek exiles from the Byzantine Empire, particularly after the conquest of Constantinople in 1452, and the expansion of mainly Venetian trading posts in the Aegean and the Greek-speaking world, had little effect at first on medicine. Only a few doctors could read Greek, and even fewer possessed Greek manuscripts. When the so-called 'collected works of Galen' were first published in 1490, they were entirely in Latin translation, and the editor of the second, 1502 edition, Hieronymus Surianus, described Galen appearing to him in a dream as a Latin author who pointed out to him corrections that were written in Latin.[136] There were a handful of exceptions in Venice, Florence, Bologna and, above all, Ferrara, where Niccolò Leoniceno and his pupils preached the superiority of Greek over Latin medicine.[137] Their first essays were primarily philological, clarifying terms in botany and medicine by showing that much incorrect Latin terminology depended on a misunderstanding or mistranslation of the original Greek. So, for example, Leoniceno in 1508 demonstrated that the opening sentences of Galen's *Art of Medicine* were not concerned with questions of logical method, as medieval commentators had believed, but with the most effective methods of teaching.[138] But their overall impact was slow in coming. The one attempt in 1500 to publish a Greek text of Galen's *Method of Healing* and his shorter *Method of Healing for Glaucon* seems to have ruined the publishers and postponed an edition of Galen's complete works in Greek for more than twenty years.[139] When new and better translations were made from the Greek, they were all, with two exceptions, of texts regularly studied in medical schools and were sometimes printed alongside the older and more fallible versions. The exceptions were Linacre's versions of *The Preservation of Health* and *The Method of Healing*, which appeared as late as 1517 and 1519.[140] No wonder that a Salzburg doctor complained in 1519 that these Italian claims for the new Galen were relatively worthless, since the average physician, who lacked Greek, did not have access to what Galen had said, and had perforce to rely on earlier handbooks based on versions now regularly denounced as prone to error.[141]

All this changed with the publication by the Aldine Press in 1525–6 of the complete works of Galen in Greek, followed immediately in 1526 by Hippocrates in Greek, and then by a series of other ancient Greek physicians such as Oribasius, Paul of Aegina and Alexander of Tralles. The Greek Galen was seen through the press by five young North European scholars, the Saxon Georg Agricola, and four from England, John Clement, Edward Wotton, Thomas Lupset and Edward Rose, all associated with Oxford, and the first two later close friends of Caius in London.[142] All, it may be assumed, were friends of Linacre, and like him, they were devoted to publicising the new Hellenic medicine. The arrival of Greek stimulated a new flow of Latin translations, often improving on the Aldine edition, which, as Erasmus complained, was full of mistakes. Although not entirely sweeping away the older Latin versions, the new translations, made by translators from many regions and published in large numbers across Western Europe, came to dominate the market. Particularly from the 1540s with the collected editions of Giunta, Farri and Froben, almost every physician had access to the Latin versions of the great Greek physician that were more extensive, more accurate and stylistically more up to date than what had been available a generation earlier.[143]

They revealed a largely new medical world, one fully in tune with the widespread belief of the so-called humanists that only by returning to the purer springs of the Classics, and in the case of medicine, to the Greek Classics, could one bring about improvement in many aspects of contemporary life, in religion, ethics and general culture[144] (Figure 6). Many of our surviving Greek medical authors had been totally unknown in the Middle Ages: although a few texts had circulated in Latin translation, the so-called 'Hippocratic Corpus' was made available for the first time only in 1525, when Fabio Calvi published his Latin translation of the Corpus, to be followed the next year by the Greek. But it was Galen that stood out, not least because of the new material that only confirmed him in his status as '*princeps medicorum*', 'prince of physicians'. For the first time, scholars had access to huge amounts of his writings on pharmacology, as well as to many of his commentaries on Hippocrates, filled with enormous learning as well as with respect for his great predecessor. There was new, or at any rate more accurate, information on Galen's therapeutics, and most important of all, on Galen's anatomy. Galen's principal textbook on anatomy, *Anatomical Procedures*, became available in the West for the first time – at least, in its first nine books, and there were rumours, reported later by Caius, below, p. 59, of the rest existing somewhere in a private library. This was supplemented by *The Opinions of Hippocrates and Plato*, Galen's exposition of human anatomy in Platonic terms, and by its Aristotelian equivalent, *The Use of Parts*. This had been available in the Middle Ages, but only in an abridged form that left out almost all the technical details of dissection.[145]

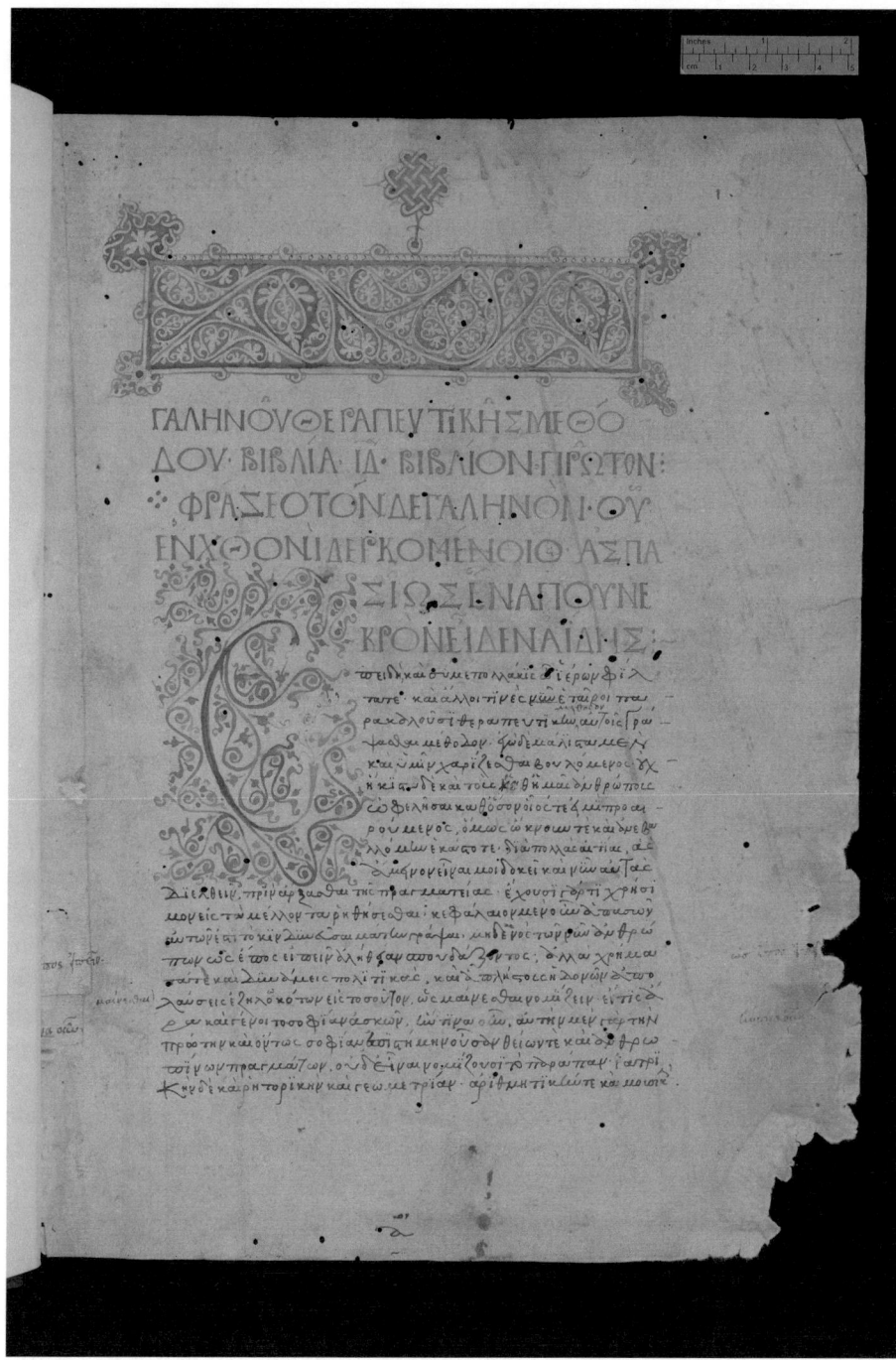

Figure 6 A Greek manuscript bought by Caius in Italy. Galen's *Method of Healing*, copied by George Tzangaropoulos, Gonville and Caius College Library, MS. 47/24, fol. 1. The second part of the work is contained in MS 355/582.

Along with other shorter texts, soon to be joined by the introductory text on *Bones*, this provided the young physicians of the 1520s and 1530s with an unprecedented understanding of anatomical dissection and its role in Galenic medicine.[146] One could for the first time appreciate the technical expertise of Galen in cutting up bodies, almost always those of animals, but there were comments, particularly in dealing with surgery, that indicated that Galen had also had some experience of cutting into human bodies. It was now clear for the first time in the West that he had insisted on the importance of regular dissection as a way of understanding the workings of the body, and demanded that true medicine depended on an accurate knowledge of bodily structures and functions. Instead of the dogmatic Galen of the Middle Ages, one had a new, more empirical investigator, full of interesting observations and ideas.[147] It was an exciting time to be a medical student or teacher as the older medicine was supplemented and in part replaced by newfound classical material from the most authoritative of all physicians.

'Anatomy' became the shibboleth of the new Galenism. What had been at best irregular and little regarded in medical schools, with the exception of Bologna and Padua, suddenly became all the rage. At Paris speeches in honour of new graduates in the 1520s make no mention of anatomy, and little of surgery: by 1537, several members of the faculty were writing or had already published their own handbooks of the new Galenic anatomy, and crowds gathered to watch Jacobus Sylvius bring already dissected limbs to illustrate his lectures on Galen.[148] There were demonstrations of anatomy in many German universities, such as Marburg and Heidelberg, while at Lutheran Wittenberg half of the lectures delivered by Philip Melanchthon on the soul, which all students had to attend, were taken up with a description of the human body according to the latest anatomical research.[149] Younger scholars, such as Vesalius, were eager to bring back the new anatomy to their own countries, and it is not surprising that Caius should have begun his lectures to the Barber-Surgeons in London shortly after his return from Italy or that in his Caius College statutes he should have made provision for two annual dissections for his medical students.[150]

A comparison of the new Galen with anatomical treatises from the Late Middle Ages is overwhelmingly in favour of the Greek physician. A medieval textbook, such as Mondino's *Anatomy*, first printed in 1478, was less extensive and less practical than the originals on which it distantly depended.[151] It explained to physicians the basic organisation of the body, stressing its purposeful functions, but conveyed little of the excitement of a Galenic dissection. Galen's injunction to every budding doctor to dissect daily was obscured, if not abolished, by the hierarchical division of activity at a formal university dissection, between a surgeon cutting the corpse, an expositor explaining to students what might be seen and how it fitted into its context, and a third person reading passages from Galen or Mondino.[152] The major weakness of the new anatomy, the sheer size of the Galenic anatomical texts on which it was based, was solved from the 1520s onwards by the production of new handbooks by authors such as Berengario da Carpi and Niccolò Massa in Italy and Johann Guinter of Andernach in Paris, which summarised Galen's conclusions and made them accessible to readers all over Europe.[153]

They also revealed that Galen was not universally infallible. Those who had the rare opportunity to examine a human body for themselves began to discover incompatibilities between the Galenic text and what they could see, but these were neither as many nor as striking as is often assumed, for most anatomical displays, whether in public or in private, involved animal dissections that served only to confirm what the sharp-eyed Galen had observed. But the greater the knowledge of human dissection, the larger the number of discrepancies. The young Andreas Vesalius, for instance, in his revision of Guinter's 1536 *Principles of Anatomy according to Galen* that he had prepared for his second course of lectures in Padua in 1538, changed approximately 15 per cent of his master's work. Far from rejecting these changes, Guinter had no hesitation in taking over almost all Vesalius' improvements into his own revision the following year, adding yet more discoveries of his own, or more likely, by his assistant, Michael Servetus.[154] Vesalius continued to dissect frequently, announcing yet further discoveries in a series of anatomical demonstrations held at Bologna in 1540 in the presence of Matteo Corti, a highly respected and highly paid Galenist. By then he had abandoned a plan for a further revision of his short handbook in favour of a major and highly innovative treatise of his own, his celebrated *De humani corporis fabrica*, published in 1543 after he had been gone from Padua for a year.[155] In it, although constantly announcing his respect for Galen, Vesalius argued that the mistakes of Galen were not sporadic, but systematic, the result of applying the results of animal dissection to the human body.

But there were others, particularly among senior scholars, who argued, like Corti, that Galen could do no wrong.[156] Vesalius' often slighting references to Galen's errors and, by implication, to those who still continued to follow him seemed to many extremely disrespectful towards those from whom he had gained much during his education. They were rightly annoyed that several passages were taken directly and unacknowledged from Galen, and that other opinions were roundly condemned although they had been until recently entirely accepted by Vesalius, and even introduced by him into his 1538 handbook. A variety of explanations were offered to explain away Galen's apparent mistakes. Jacobus Sylvius in Paris argued that it was the human body that had changed over the centuries, and hence that Galen's description was accurate for his own day, although how many followed him in this view is unclear.[157] Others, particularly those who were involved in editing or translating Galen, put the blame on Vesalius' weak understanding of Greek. Janus Cornarius (1500–58), a contentious opponent of Vesalius, was so angry that he struck out the name of Vesalius from his own copy of his revised versions of Galen with such force that the imprint can be seen clearly today even through several pages.[158] Caius, who had worked on fragmentary portions of Galen's anatomical works in Greek while staying with Vesalius, pointed out many errors in Vesalius' translation both in his own Latin versions and commentaries and in the notes he later added in their margins.[159] Vesalius, or Wesalius as Caius continued to call him in private, acknowledged the strength of some of his criticisms, taking them over into the second edition of the *Fabrica* in 1555.[160] But textual criticism and improved translation technique could do only so much, and by the end of the century, except in Spain under the baleful influence of the *protomedico* Luis Mercado (1520–1606), Galenic anatomy was supplemented, if not superseded, by that of Vesalius and his successors.[161]

Caius' interest in ancient anatomy did not stop with Galen, but involved him in an unusual and, for medicine at least, unique enterprise, the reconstruction of what he believed to be a 'lost' ancient text, the book on anatomy written by the father of medicine, Hippocrates. His description of his methods and what he claimed to have achieved takes up several pages in his *Autobibliography*, pp. 70–72, written up at length since he had not otherwise published his discovery earlier. By doing so, he could follow Galen in taking anatomical investigation back to the earliest years of Greek medicine and establish a pedigree that confirmed its status as an essential part of the medical art. Whatever might be thought of Galen's anatomy, there could now be little doubt that proper dissection and recording of information went back to none other than Hippocrates, and Caius was rightly proud of his find. That modern scholarship has dismissed his claim, like so much else in his writings, should not disguise his ingenuity, the ancient documentation that he used in his reconstruction or the remarkable methodology that he adopted. Only a man of considerable learning such as Caius could have attempted such a task.

The account given by Caius makes it clear that he took his inspiration from Galen, who had argued, on grounds that are far from convincing today, that Hippocrates had practised dissection and thus provided him with a convincing precedent for his own activities. It was a claim that he made in passing in a variety of treatises, notably *The Opinions of Hippocrates and Plato*, in which he tried to show that his own description of the human body and its workings agreed with what these two great figures had written five hundred years previously. In *My own Books* and elsewhere he referred to a treatise in six books he had written on Hippocrates' anatomy, which is now lost.[162] The title is ambiguous, for it could indicate a general survey of anatomical information within the Hippocratic writings or, more specifically, as Caius took it, a commentary on a book of this title. One such book indeed exists within the Hippocratic Corpus and was made available to Western scholars for the first time in print in 1525–6. But it was also obvious that this tiny tract, a mere page and a half long in the standard nineteenth-century edition of Littré, could not have been all that Galen had read, for his comments covered aspects of the body not mentioned there.[163] Caius was also aware from his own reading of Galen, as he explains in his *Autobibliography*, that the numbers and titles assigned to ancient treatises, even by their authors, were not fixed, and that parts of writings by one author could well become separated, circulating on their own or becoming attached to works by others. This was something that Galen and many of his Hellenistic predecessors had touched upon in their Hippocratic commentaries, and encouraged Caius in his search for the lost work.[164] He found it in a group of small treatises, *Glands, The Heart, The Nature of Bones*, like *Anatomy*, all unknown in the West before 1525–6, which, with the addition of an introductory passage from *Leverage*, could be put together in a coherent and, to Caius, sensible order to produce the original *Anatomy*. It was an ingenious, unusual and from the point of view of the methodology involved, exemplary suggestion. It was also deeply flawed, for although there might be connections between *Glands, The Nature of Bones* and *Anatomy*, short texts possibly dating from around 400 B.C., *The Heart* is at least a century later and written in a different style and context.[165] Like much of Caius' historical writing in general, he reaches an improbable conclusion on the basis of documentation whose problems neither he nor any of his contemporaries fully understood.[166]

If the new anatomy, whether in its Galenic or later Vesalian manifestation, can be considered one of the most important changes in medicine during the Renaissance, its impact on medical practice is harder to determine.[167] Most physicians did not have the time, the interest or the expertise to carry out dissection themselves, let alone pursue a plan of research such as Galen had recommended. They were content with the new handbooks, supplemented by printed collections of images, which confirmed the general truths of Galenic medicine. Luis Mercado and others in Spain may have been ultra-conservative in demanding a return to the anatomy described in Galen's *The Use of Parts*, but they had their reasons: Vesalian descriptive anatomy was not as useful to the physician as Galen's own writing because it said very little about the function and purpose that were, in Mercado's view, essential for the understanding of the workings of the body in sickness and health.[168]

Far more significant for the physicians of the mid-sixteenth century was the abundance of new observations and ideas revealed in the newly published Galenic texts. Galen, as writers like Julius Alexandrinus (1506–1590) and Andreas Laguna (1499–1560) pointed out, was by no means as consistent as he claimed to be, and his apparent self-contradictions offered much space for new interpretations within an overall Galenic framework.[169] The constant debates among physicians, as well as the relative ease with which alternative ideas, even some of those associated from the 1550s onwards with the Paracelsians, could be assimilated were signs of strength, not of weakness, as Ian Maclean has shown.[170] Besides, Renaissance physicians had a new sense of what constituted effective medical practice, the proper application of 'method'. As we have seen, above, p. 31, the vigorous debate in the thirteenth and fourteenth centuries over the meaning of 'method' in terms of logical analysis had been shown by Leoniceno to rest on a misunderstanding of Galen, whose view of how a physician should proceed was far wider than that.

Late medieval Galenism had privileged diagnosis from taking the pulse and examining urine above a full physical examination, and many physicians had gained a reputation also for their use of astrology or horoscopic medicine to forecast and to control the course of an illness. The publication in 1536 of a treatise on medical 'astronomy' ascribed to Galen appeared to strengthen this practice, but it was pushed to the fringes of acceptable medicine by the discovery of Galen's general disdain for astrology and of his insistence that pulse and urine were not enough by themselves to establish an effective diagnosis.[171] Instead, he had demanded close observation of everything concerning the patient, as well as, if possible, his or her normal state of health. Only after this could one begin to proceed to diagnosis and treatment, both requiring careful judgment of many subtleties as well as an organised method. Galen had set out his own method in the fourteen books of his *Method of Healing*, and in the two-book version that he had dedicated to Glaucon. The latter was short enough to be the subject of commentary as far back as Late Antiquity, and remained popular down to the seventeenth century. Its brevity, however, required to be supplemented and its concise formulations explained by a teacher, and in the second quarter of the sixteenth century there was no better guide than Da Monte at Padua.[172] The larger book, although translated into Latin in the Middle Ages and available in print from 1490 in the version of Gerard of Cremona (d. 1187), remained largely the preserve of a few experts until the publication of Linacre's version in 1519, after which it was regarded as Galen's most important work on therapeutics.[173]

Over the course of his teaching career in Padua, which lasted from 1539 until his death in 1552, Da Monte lectured on the main standard texts of theoretical and practical medicine, including Galen's *Method of Healing, for Glaucon* and on his *Art of Medicine*.[174] His erudition was considerable, and he possessed a celebrated acquaintance with all the works of Galen in both Greek and Latin. He also had the ability to select and to inform his students with clarity and at times humour how they should proceed in their encounters with patients. His visits to the bedside, often accompanied by colleagues and students, involved both exposition and discussion of potential therapies.[175] His reputation brought students from around Europe to hear and see him in action in Padua. He had two weaknesses. His desire to derive the utmost information from the texts in front of him, coupled with his prodigious learning, meant that he rarely covered all that he wished to say in a single lecture or in the whole course: over-diligent copyists recorded his apologies for breaking off his exposition prematurely before reaching the end.[176] His second weakness, if that is what it can be called, was a reluctance or inability to publish himself. He was not alone in this, for the process of preparing lectures for printing was (and is) tedious, and students became used to taking down his words exactly so as to have them for reference when they returned home. Only a portion of his lectures appeared during his lifetime, but after his death, several former students issued their transcripts of his lectures and his consultations, taking care not to claim authorship for themselves.

Caius, a former student of Da Monte, while on his way home to England, handed over to the Basle publishers Froben and Episcopius the two books of his *Method of Healing according to the Princes of Medicine, Galen of Pergamum and Giambattista Da Monte of Verona.*[177] This is an ambiguous title, disguising exactly what Caius owed to Galen or his old teacher. Although Da Monte is praised along with Galen in the preface, there is no indication that this book had been derived in large part from Da Monte's lectures, as Caius admits, below, p. 56.[178] The second printing of the work, by Bergagne at Louvain in 1556, omits Da Monte's name entirely and is accompanied by a variety of shorter works by Caius. It was this failure to acknowledge properly the role of Da Monte that seems to have annoyed another student of his, Johann Crato von Crafftheim (1519–1585). Crato had overlapped very briefly with Caius in Padua and went on to have a distinguished medical and diplomatic career as one of the doctors of the Holy Roman Emperor.[179] He seems to have been close to Da Monte and took it upon himself to see through the press a variety of his works that had been left in manuscript. In 1555 Crato published his own version of Da Monte's lectures at Basle under a very similar title, *The Method of Healing according to Galen and Giambattista Da Monte of Verona*, stressing in its preface the extent to which it derived from his teacher's lectures.[180] In letters, and in other publications bearing on an appropriate method for use in healing, Crato further emphasised his dependence on Da Monte, and by implication, the deceit by Caius.[181]

Caius' defence takes up two and a half folios of the *Autobibliography*, listing instances both ancient and modern where authors 'borrowed' in various ways from their sources, sometimes with express acknowledgment, sometimes not. Not everyone will be convinced by the comparison between his own actions and Vergil's use of Homer, Oribasius' long citations of Galen or Erasmus' collection of aphorisms taken from earlier writers, for, certainly in the second edition of 1556, it is difficult to find even a minimal allusion to the involvement of Da Monte. Nor is his argument convincing that by failing to mention Da Monte he was performing a service to Galen, the ultimate source of Da Monte, for by doing this he was implicitly accusing his teacher of the same crime that Crato attributed to him. He might have done better to point out more clearly the differences between his productions and those of Crato. The two works were not identical, and indeed, were reprinted together as if sufficiently dissimilar in a two-volume edition of Da Monte's *Opuscula*, curated by Girolamo Donzellini at Basle in 1558.[182]

The medicine that Caius brought back to Britain was an elite medicine, fully in tune with the ideas and aspirations of the London College, whose statutes, whether as revised by Edward Wotton as president in 1541–42 or by Caius himself a little later in 1555, demanded a detailed knowledge of

all the works of Hippocrates and Galen.[183] This medicine stressed the importance of the individual patient's balance of humours, while at the same time
it was capable of dealing with a relatively new epidemic such as the Sweat.
The great names in medicine of the period were all Galenists, some like Jean
Fernel (1497–1558) writing large syntheses, others, like Girolamo Mercuriale (1530–1606), collecting information from a wide variety of classical
texts to create original studies of epidemiology, children's diseases or sports
medicine.[184] Israel Spach's 1597 collection of ancient gynaecological writings became a standard source for women's diseases, while the 39 books of
Observations and Cures by Pieter van Foreest (1522–1597) furnish a remarkable account of the practice of a learned physician in France and in the Netherlands.[185] It was by no means closed to new interpretations. The so-called
Paris Hippocratics used their commentaries on the 'new' Hippocratic texts
to criticise many aspects of Galen, while still retaining his overall framework. Girolamo Fracastoro's studies of contagious diseases contained much
shrewd observation as well as novel ideas on the spread of epidemic disease, while a glance at the published collection of letters exchanged between
Crato von Crafftheim and his friends in Italy and Germany shows both the
vigour of contemporary medical debates and the eagerness with which distant recipients awaited the latest contribution to Europe-wide controversies.
As Ian Maclean has argued, it is only in the light of later developments that
the Renaissance Galenists have come to be seen as dyed-in-the-wool con-
servatives. They themselves were convinced with some justice that the new
material from the past allowed them to go far beyond what their medieval
predecessors had done, constantly offering new possibilities that would help
towards therapy.[186]

It is true that Galenism was being challenged, most notably in Germany
and, to a lesser extent, in London, from the late 1550s onwards by the rise of
Paracelsian medicine. The *Annals of the College of Physicians* are filled with
accounts of proceedings against those who denied the authority of Galen (several of whom were later admitted to the college), and many leading Protestant
magnates supported unorthodox practitioners. But among the elite, advo-
cates of Paracelsian theory were few in number, and Galenists, most notably
Gessner and Johann Guinter, quickly found ways of adapting for their own
purposes many of the therapies the Paracelsians championed. Gessner's *The
Treasure of Euonymus, 'conteyninge the wonderfull hid secretes of nature,
touchinge the most apte formes to prepare and destyl medicines, for the conservation of health,'* originally printed in Latin at Zurich in 1552 by Andreas
Gessner and Rudolf Weissenbach, was a European best-seller.[187] By the time
it appeared in English in 1559, translations into German, French and Italian
were already on the market. It showed that remedies such as 'quintessence,
aurum potabile, hippocras, aromatic wines, balms, oils, perfumes, garnish-
ing waters' and the like were perfectly compatible with traditional teaching.
As distinguished a Galenist as Vesalius' old teacher in Paris, Johann Guinter,

saw nothing strange in producing a large work in two volumes, showing how the old and new medicine could be reconciled.[188] Others also published their own syntheses.

Renaissance Galenism was thus a flexible system of medicine, based on methodical observation and reasoning, and as effective as, and arguably less dangerous than, other types of medicine on offer. It also depended on a close rapport between patient and physician, and the amount of wealth that Caius amassed during his lifetime from his practice shows that rich patients were more than satisfied with the treatments that he offered them. His continental training and his expertise in anatomy, as well as his abundant learning (both within and without medicine) will all have contributed to confirming that here was a physician who shared their intellectual interests, whom they could trust, and who had a sound record of success.

Notes

1 Jebb (1729: viii–xv), also emphasising its value for any future biographer.
2 Beroaldo (1487: sig. a.ii.r 1500): *Interpres inuolucra explicat: obscura illustrat: arcana reuelat: & quod ille strictim & quasi transeunter attingit: hic copiose & diligenter enodat. . . . ipsi interpretes honorandi quorum lucubrationes etiam posteris prosunt,* a reference I owe to Paul Gwynne.
3 McNair (1969), sceptical of a direct connection; Traister (2004), Caius played as a comic character; Traister (2015), Caius as emblematic of the medical profession; Pettigrew (2007: 57), a name deliberately adopted by a quack; Armitage (2009), a satire on Caius himself.
4 For praise of Caius by others, see below, p. 123 Abraham Fleming; p. 113, note 12, Ole Worm; p. 110 Johann Rode. Nutton (1987) was the first to draw attention to his work on Galenic manuscripts.
5 Venn (1912); Raven (1947: 138–49); Clark (1964: I, 106–24); Brooke (1985: 55–79); Nutton (2004a); Cagliuso (2015).
6 Below, p. 54. Stiward (1491–1571), a mercer, an alderman from 1526, thrice mayor, and twice a member of parliament for Norwich, was a major figure in the city from the 1520s until his death, Virgoe (1982). Fay (2015: 139–40) suggests a possible link between Caius' views on epidemics and some of the practical reforms carried out by Stiward.
7 Crankshaw and Gillespie (2011).
8 Grafton (2017). Venn (1912: 53) notes the report that Caius had a considerable share in the composition of Richard Grafton's 1569 *Chronicle.*
9 Venn (1912: 36–8); Brook (1985: 75–7).
10 Below, pp. 54–55: Caius 1570c 2r–3v = 70–2 R.; 1552: 6–7 = 6–7 R.
11 Knighton (2004).
12 Caius (1552: 6 = 7 R.) wrongly gives his name as Thirtle. John Thixtill, another Norfolk man, was a Fellow of Pembroke from 1515. His will of 1541 describes him as "of Newport Pond, Essex, and St Botolph, Cambridge", (Venn and Venn 1922: 220). Caius may have misremembered the name or the printer misread his handwriting. For Skippe, previously Master of Caius, see Brooke (1985: 49–51); Newcombe (2004).
13 For these individuals, see Woolfson (2004), with Caius 1544b: II, 4; Bowker (2004c); Archer (2004); Sowerby (2010).

14   Venn (1912: 5), citing Caius' note in a Hebrew Bible, Ms. 404/625. For his early theological writings, see below, p. 54. Fragments of patristic authors are included in his miscellaneous MS 355/582, viii–ix.
15   Caius (1574c: 91–7 = 74–8 R.).
16   The dates of his arrival and matriculation at Padua are not certain, as the relevant archives are lost. The document of 15 June 1541 printed by Venn (1912: 55) was typical of those given to students leaving Padua after graduation, confirming their earlier matriculation and granting them freedom from charges on themselves and their belongings at the customs on their way home.
17   Brooke (1985: 56).
18   Caius (1557); Pollard and Bakewell (2004).
19   Caius (1544; pref., p. 5); Dowling (1997): Martin and Davies (2004).
20   Fletcher (1977); Lewis (1977).
21   London, Wellcome Library, classmark EPB 56, 3933, 5242, 5280, all of 1527.
22   Caius (1556), dedicatory preface, p. 135, dated January 1556: Kitsch (2004).
23   Maddison, Pelling and Webster (1977); Nutton (2004c).
24   Both men provided him with information on manuscripts, see Nutton (1987a: 59–61, 84–5). For Wotton, see Pollard and Wallis (2004), and for a re-evaluation of his copy of the Galenic commentary on the Hippocratic *Regimen in Acute Diseases*, Pietrobelli (forthcoming 1).
25   For Clement (d. 1572), Wenkebach (1925) provides a mine of information in his notes; Gundert (2006); Wallis (2004). Caius later loaned his own copy of Dionysius the Areopagite to Clement, but it was never returned, Grierson (1978: 520).
26   Reed (1925: 26) published a partial inventory of Clement's London library in 1549–50, which can be supplemented by recent discoveries. Dr Grantley MacDonald is preparing a major study of Clement and his library.
27   The delicate Anglo-French political situation discouraged study by Englishmen in Paris, long the leading medical school in Northern Europe, although its reputation in the 1530s was not as high as it was to become only a few years later.
28   Ongaro (1981: 75–134); Grendler (2002: 32–3).
29   Ongaro (1981: 118–26, 1994); Muccillo (1986).
30   Vesalius (1538); Singer and Rabin (1946); Kusukawa (2012: 185–90); Nutton (2017c).
31   Guinter and Vesalius (1538); Nutton (2017a).
32   Nutton (2017a), who includes a transcription and discussion of Vesalius' notes. For Vesalius and the *Fabrica*, O'Malley (1964); Garrison and Hast (2014).
33   O'Malley (1955).
34   Fortuna (2012).
35   Leoniceno (1492).
36   Pietrobelli (forthcoming 2) suggests that rather than composing a specific volume of conjectures, Agricola inserted his many corrections into the margins of his copy of the Aldine.
37   Nutton (1987a: 39–42); Galen (1538: II A2r; IV *2r), with Gundert (2006, 2009: 154–5, 171–4); Gärtner (2015: 173–6, 186–8). The intermediary was probably the Basle scholar Simon Grynaeus, who stayed with Thomas More in London in 1531.
38   Boudon-Millot (2007: CCVI–VIII). For Caius' use of Donzellini's modern Latin translation of Galen's *Barley Gruel* to fill in a lacuna, see below, p. 98, n. 141.
39   EtonAdv I, 196–97: "Should someone wish to restore the Greek by reference to the Latin translations (which I see many today boast of doing), how grievously would he be deceived." (*Si quis igitur ad latinas transl. graeca velit restituere, id quod multos hodie iactitare video, quam egregie deciperetur!*)

40 EtonAdv: I, front page: *is me dotavit et ego illum.*
41 Galen (1541–1545, 1541–1542). The slightly later Basle editor, Hieronymus Gemusaeus, relied less on manuscripts for his edition of the Latin *Opera omnia*, Basle: Hieronymus Froben and Nicolaus Episcopius, 1542, than on conjecture., see Hieronymus (2005: no. 054).
42 His linguistic expertise was commended by his teacher Guinter in all his editions of the *Institutiones* (1536, 32r; Basle, 1539: sig vʳ), and he continued to be praised for his work as a translator by Galenists long after the publication of the *Fabrica*. For his relations with Gadaldino, see the preface to Galen (1541: 1, 3).
43 For Gadaldino, see Garofalo (2004). In his collations of *The Dissection of Nerves*, EtonAdv. I, 204, Caius also made use of the variant readings assembled by Gadaldino in Galen, but "not religiously or for the entire book".
44 De Lacy (1978: 31); Nutton (1987a); Boudon-Millot (2007: 71–9); Gundert (2009: 173–4); Gärtner (2015: 188–90). The Latin word Caius uses to describe his work as editor is '*castigare*', see below, p. 105, note 216.
45 Below, pp. 70–72. He was following Galen's practice in dealing with Hippocratic writings, but this precedent should not detract from his achievements.
46 Caius (1556: 181 = 91 R). For Caius' interest in brewing, see now Funk (2016).
47 Exactly when he was appointed is unclear, as is the title of his post. In 1555 and below p. 66, he describes his post as that of lecturing on the teachings of Aristotle in Greek, presumably in the academic year 1542–3. His 'customs' certificate of June 1541 describes him as lecturing in Greek, while the degree certificate of May 1541 calls him professor of Greek dialectic, i.e. Aristotle, see Venn (1912: 55, 57). His own copy of Aristotle, Basle: Bebel, 1531, Caius College Library, sig. G.32.4.5, bears many early notes by Caius. A later fellow of Caius College wrongly believed that he had taught medicine at Padua, R. Parker (ob. 1624), Gonville and Caius College, MS 94/173. p. 34 = MS 361/592, p. 22.
48 For Knolles (d. 1583), diplomat and MP, see Woolfson (1998; 248–9); Caius (1544b: II, 4).
49 Crato (1555). For Crato's role in publishing Da Monte's manuscripts after his death, see Hieronymus (2005: nos. 388–92).
50 Compare the contemporary journey of Jean Matal around many of the same Italian libraries, Hobson (1975).
51 Nutton (1987a). What he reports of his findings in his notes and what he says here do not always correspond.
52 For memories of Venice elsewhere, see Caius 1570b: 5r, 20v = 30, 50 R.; the Rubicon,1570b: 27v = 60 R. At EtonAdv III, 501 = IV, 18 K., he mentions the death of a Pole who broke his neck when falling from his horse at Padua.
53 Bosman-Jelgersma (1996a, b); Santing (2010).
54 His medical Greek MSS included Gonville and Caius MSS 47/24 (Galen); 50/27 (Hippocrates); 76/43 (Actuarius and Galen); 77/44 (Alexander of Tralles and Rhazes); 355/582 (Galen and Hippocrates); 360/587 (Galen) Late Alexandrian philosophical commentators are included in MSS 495/264 (Proclus and Syrianus); 500/382 (Simplicius).
55 Nutton (1987a); Boudon-Millot (2007: 71–9). See, for the list of his editions and collations, below, pp. 82–4.
56 E.g. Caius 1544: 4v "An outstanding doctor, without parallel in Europe"; EtonAdv I, 334: "An old book belonging to the most learned John Clement gave me the opportunity for this emendation."
57 Boudon-Millot (2007: ccxxxx–xxxvii); Guardasole (2010); Gärtner (2015: 186–90).
58 Woolfson (1998); Nutton (2011).

59 As Tony Grafton has pointed out in an unpublished lecture, there is no direct evidence of a personal meeting, although Caius' lament for Gessner might imply this, and the fact that Gessner did not acquire his copy of the 1544 *Methodus medendi* until a year or so later may be a possible indication that theirs could have been an entirely epistolary friendship. Cf. below, p. 79, for epistolary friendships with Melanchthon and Camerarius.

60 Serrai (1990: especially 312, 316, 324–6); Delisle (2008); Leu (2016a, b); Leu and Ruoss (2016).

61 He was paid 15 Pfund for this by the publishers (Leu 2016a: 96).

62 A list of Caius' books is printed in Gessner (1555: 59v–60r).

63 Funk (2017) discusses Caius' contributions to Gessner's *Historia animalium*.

64 Gessner (1560a: 6, 15, 25–8, 37–8, 48, 55, 72–3, 1560b: 80). Caius' contributions were later brought together and printed by Seres along with the *Autobibliography* in 1570. For newly discovered drawings sent by Caius, see Egmond (2013, 2016).

65 Gessner (1577: 133v–37v); cf. f. 115r. A long letter of Caius is incorporated in Gessner (1551–58: 4: 1294–6). See also Funk (2017).

66 Delisle (2008: 215), for the editorial process, noting that Gessner kept an annotated copy of this letter in his files. For Caius' book, below, p. 101, note 181.

67 Serrai (1990: 339–48); Leu (2016a: 256–8). The book was Valerius Cordus, *Annotationes in Dioscoridem*, Strasbourg: J. Rihel, 1561, which contains several other treatises by Cordus, as well as Gessner's own *De hortis Germaniae*. By 1565 (Gessner 1577: 111v–12v) Gessner believed that Caius now intended to send everything to Froben, see below, note 78.

68 Despite Gessner's hopes, a revised edition was never published. For the posthumous publication of some of Caius' contributions to Gessner's books, see Funk (2017).

69 For traces of other letters sent by Caius to Gessner, see Gessner (1560a: 37, 72–5); Raven (1947: 148).

70 Delisle (2008). For the wider context, see Findlen (1994).

71 For Parkhurst, see Gessner (1577: 134v), and for his experiences in London when delivering a letter he had brought from Gessner to Caius, see Venn (1912: 10). Turner was the recipient from Gessner (1562) of a long letter on his own books: for his relationship with Gessner in general, see Jones (1988b: 16, 91–3). For Gessner's comments on Edward Wotton, see Nutton (1985a).

72 Gessner (1577: 136v), although Gessner does not seem entirely sure whether Bullock had gone back to Paris or was now in Italy, and when, or if, he would return from Italy. For Bullock, see Rex (2004a).

73 Grierson (1978: 516, nos. 70–3).

74 Gessner (1560a: 3–6), with also a long poem in Greek.

75 Gessner (1553: 2). The original preface was reprinted at the back of the 1560 edition. For the wider context of Gessner's dedications, see Blair (2017). The importance of Zurich at this point for English Protestants is well brought out by McCullough (2017: 323–30).

76 Stevenson (1866: 10, no. 17, dated March 7, 1561). Gessner (1560a: 3) mentions that the Grey brothers had died before the book reached them, and refers (1560a: 6) to Cecil's own interest in natural history. Bishop Parkhurst had originally encouraged Gessner to dedicate the second edition to Elizabeth, for which he was thanked in the preface to the 1560 *Icones avium* (Blair 2017: 184).

77 Leu (2016a: 179).

78 Welti (1964: 145–51) discusses Caius' relations with Oporinus and Froben. In a letter of 1565 (Gessner 1577: 111v–12v) Gessner told his nephew Zwinger that

Caius was about to send his book on British dogs (among others) to Froben and Episcopius: if they did not want them, he wished them to be passed on to Gessner.

79 Raven (1947: 139). Caius' statement, below, pp. 79–80, that he decided to investigate pronunciation only after beginning his autobibliography would also seem to rule out a visit before 1543.

80 Moore (1918: 416–17).

81 Respectively Caius 1570b: 7v, 13v–14v, 24v, 25v, 26r and 29v = pp. 34, 42, 56, 57, 58, 63 R. Hugh Owen (1825: I, 345–7) rightly doubted Caius' presence in Shrewsbury (Caius 1552: 10 = 11 R; 1555: 128 = 66 R); as also did Charles Creighton (1891: I, 259). Venn (1912: 8) posits a brief visit. In a note in his copy of Gessner's *Icones*, Gonville and Caius College Library, L. 19.4, p. 58, he reports seeing a massive set of reindeer horns while visiting a noble patient in Kent in 1554,

82 For patients, see Venn (1912: 8, n. 1), and for his links with London antiquarians, Grafton (2017). A note in his copy of Aristotle, Gonville and Caius College Library, G.32.5, fol. 205v, records that Thomas Wyntersale, a servant of Lady Copley, could move his ears in all directions.

83 For Cecil and his family, below, p. 65; and for the Bacons, below, p. 65. A hint that he was not a royal physician may be found in his *Annals of the College of Physicians*: 59 R., where he notes that Robert Huyck had to step down as President in 1564 because of his commitments as a Royal Physician. If Caius had been dismissed in disgrace before then, it is hard to believe he would have played such an important part in the royal visit to Cambridge of 1564, or that his college would have been allowed to play host to Elizabeth's ladies in waiting.

84 Clark (1964) is the standard account.

85 Maddison et al. (1977).

86 Clark (1964: 106–24). A note at EtonAdv V, 41 = XV, 440 K., probably from the late 1550s, compares Galen's complaint at popular support for astrologers with his own day (*"ita nostro tempore"*).

87 He was one of the three fellows who wrote to Cambridge University in 1554, successfully warning against granting a medical degree to Simon Ludford, an apothecary, *Annals*, 29–33 R; Clark (1964: 112–14). The original letters to the university are in British Library, MS Sloane 3562, 59r–64r.

88 Brooke (1985: 53–70); Nickson (2005).

89 Some, no doubt, he retained for self-keeping in his room, where they were destroyed in 1572, below, p. 115. Ceri Law pointed out to me that, given the queen's own preference for a more Catholic ceremonial than her bishops wished, it was not foolish in the 1560s to hope for some restoration of older ceremonies, and hence to refrain from disposing of vestments and the like.

90 Caius (1904); the *Annals* of the College of Physicians are printed in Roberts (1912).

91 Venn (1912: 74); Caius (1568); rev. ed. 1574a = Roberts (1912); Plomer (1926–27).

92 Caius (1574c) = Roberts (1912); Nutton (2017b). Some of it may go back to a document presented to Queen Elizabeth on her visit to Cambridge in 1564 (Venn 1912: 54).

93 E.g. his claims for Norwich (via Polydore Vergil) or his account of Brennus (via Geoffrey of Monmouth). His etymologies contain a similar blend of ingenuity and impossibility. He was particularly interested in the early sections of Polydore Vergil, to judge from his annotations in his copy, Caius College Library, F.3.10.

94 Grafton (2017).

95 Venn (1912: 50).

96 Caius (1904: 90).

97 Caius (1574d: 3 = 3 R.).

98 Given the context, the latter interpretation is more likely, although it requires the change to '*Gallicum*', and save for the name of the disease as '*morbus Gallicus*', no example has yet been found of its use by itself to denote a sufferer. For his possible work on the University Statutes, see Venn (1912: 53).

99 Michael Prichard suggests that much of his conflict with the fellows resulted from their failure to live up to his high standards, particularly in matters of financial administration.

100 Compare Caius' denunciation of the lifestyle of the wealthy in his *Sweating Sicknesse* (1552: 19, 22 = 19, 21 R.), as well as his condemnation of modern life in his *Annals* (1904: 83) and *History* (1574c: 3, 91–5 = 3, 74–7 R.). The age difference between him and his junior fellows, let alone students, will have sharpened his sense of authority, which was exercised equally forcefully by other heads of houses.

101 Nutton (2011).

102 Caius (1574d: 3–5 = 4–5 R.).

103 Below, p. 101.

104 For a detailed discussion of his religious views in the context of the 1560s and 1570s, see below, Appendix II.

105 Venn (1912: 32–3, 53–4). His contribution was not entirely a success as his high, squeaky voice was at times inaudible, and the queen had to leave her seat to come close enough to hear him. For his further involvement in university affairs, see Law (2018).

106 For Cecil and his family, see below, p. 65, and at *History* 132 = p. 106 R.

107 Venn (1912: 53); Grafton (2017) suggests that the book on the antiquity of Cambridge depended on work done by others in Parker's circle.

108 Porter (1958: 209), suggesting that in 1570 half the university might have been sympathetic to Caius' views; Law (2018, ch. 6). For the wider context, McGrath (1967: 47–99, labelling the period 1558–1570 as "the years of uncertainty"); Walsham (1999: 20), (2014: 53–102). Cf. Strype (1821: 155), attributing Caius' views on Greek pronunciation to his popery.

109 The letter of complaint dated by Venn (1912: 26) to 1565 is redated by Grierson (1978: 524, note 10) to 1572/3.

110 For the belief of an anonymous annotator that the Queen had ordered the archbishop to cut his ties with Caius, see below, p. 122.

111 For Gessner, see below, pp. 73–6; for Caius' will and Linacre (Venn 1912: 77, 74).

112 For traces of his lost works, see Appendix I.

113 Cf. Caius' preface (1552: 3 = p. 4 R.), describing the Latin version of the treatise on the Sweat as being aimed at 'men of lernynge more at large'.

114 Below p. 79. An English audience would also have noticed the range and importance of the names of the political and social elite Caius chose to mention.

115 Caius may have used the version of the *Catalogus omnium lucubrationum*, published by Froben at Basle in 1537, rather than any earlier printing. An accessible edition of the various versions is provided by Allen (1906–1958: I, Ep. 1, 1–46).

116 Gessner (1545: 136–42; 1577: 133v–137v).

117 Simler (1566).

118 Grierson (1978: 514); Lycosthenes and J. Simler (Gessner 1555: 36r–v). We cannot tell what books were lost in 1572 or still remained in Cambridge at Caius' death.

119 The discovery of the Vlatadon MS, which contains a complete text of the treatise, has outdated all previous editions and translations before the edition by

Boudon-Millot (2007: 134–73). *Slander* is mentioned, p. 170. For *Prognosis*, see Nutton (1979); and for *My own Opinions*, Nutton (1999).

120 Cardano (1663: 1, 55–9); Maclean (1999). The 1557 edition (Cardano 1663: 1, 60–95; Maclean 2004: 169) expands the title to *De libris propriis eorumque ordine et usu*, combining two Galenic titles. The list of books constitutes chap. 45 in the 1663 edition (Maclean 2004: 381–91; tr. Stoner 1931: 99–100).

121 Siraisi (1997: 9, 25–6, 233, n. 14).

122 The recommendation for the archbishop is reported at length in Cardano, *Consilia* 22 (1663, 9, 123–52); and summarised in English in Wykes (1969: 133–5); Fierz (1983: 16–21). Aquilecchia (1999: 385, 389) is cautious about his lodging with Cheke, although the two men had been acquainted since 1549 (Cardano 1663: 5, 512). For Caius' acquaintance with Cheke, note the marginal reference to an opinion of Cheke's in Caius' own copy of the 1531 Aristotle, Caius College Library G.32.5, fol. 165r.

123 Cardano (1663: 5, 503–8), with a typically revised version of the earlier horoscope.

124 Galen, *Anatomical Procedures* I,i: II, 217 K.; *My own Books* 3, 9, with Boudon-Millot (2007: 198–200).

125 Raiola (2015).

126 Caius (1552: 4–7 = pp. 5–8 R.).

127 Haddon (1567).

128 Below, p. 58, with the notes, pp. 89–91; O'Malley (1955).

129 Gessner (1577: 133v–37v).

130 Nutton (2009: 220–2), showing that Gessner was not the only scholar to present Galen as an ethical paragon.

131 The detailed description of the complex metres used by Framingham, omitted from the earlier description (Caius, 1552: 5 = 7 R.) also confirms both men's credentials as Latinists. See also Waquet (2001).

132 For Guinter (1505–1574) see above, p. 35; Nutton (2017a: esp. 22–7).

133 One non-medical scholar who appreciated Caius' work was Gian Vincenzo Pinelli (1535–1601), see the letters exchanged with Charles Dupuy (Raugei 2001: 242–9, 274, 279, who is unaware of another letter exchanged between them on the topic, Munich, Bayerische Staatsbibliothek, CLM 10364, n. 562).

134 Agrimi and Crisciani (1988); Siraisi (1990).

135 Boudon-Millot (2007: CCVI–VIII); Fortuna (2005); Agrimi and Crisciani (1994).

136 Galen (1502: pref); Nutton (1987a: 21–3); Fortuna (2005: 473–5).

137 Leoniceno (1492); Mugnai Carrara (1991).

138 Leoniceno (1508). First printed as an appendix to his *In libros Galeni e greca in linguam latinam a se translatos*, Venice: J. Pentius de Leucho, and often reprinted along with his translation of the *Art of Medicine*.

139 Nutton (1987a: 28–9).

140 Galen, *De sanitate tuenda*, tr. T. Linacre. Paris: D. Mattheu for G. Hittorp 1517; *Methodus medendi*. Paris: D. Mattheu for G. Hittorp 1519.

141 Leonhard Schmaus in a letter of 24 September 1519 to Joachim Vadianus (Arbenz 1891: 248). For Schmaus, Bonorand (1980: 200–1).

142 Wenkebach (1925: 14–17, 52–5); Nutton (1987a); Pietrobelli (2013); for the date, Potter (1998).

143 Durling (1961); Fortuna (2005).

144 Typical statements include Jason Pratensis (1486–1558) (1527: sig. A5r): 'Without Greek all our profession is an imposture'; and S. Singkeler (d. 1547) (1537: pref.): 'Those who have no linguistic skills cannot break the shell and are cheated of the nut.'

145 French (1979); Nutton (2008b). A better version by Niccolò da Reggio appears to have been rarely copied or used.
146 Garofalo and Debru (2005). In general Rocca (2008).
147 Rocca (2003: 208).
148 Nutton (2017a: 18–22).
149 Helm (2001); for Spain, Skaarup (2015).
150 Venn (1912: 9), also noting the reference to Caius as an anatomist on his 1564 College portrait.
151 Mondino (1992).
152 French (1999); Nutton (2017a).
153 Berengario (1521, 1522); Massa (1536); Nutton (2017a). The translations in Lind (1975) remain fundamental.
154 Nutton (2017a); Guinter (1539) is an improvement on what Vesalius himself had written in 1538, particularly in its discussion of the nerves and veins in the legs.
155 Eriksson (1959); Vesalius (1543). For the date, above, p. 35; for the aborted plans for a third edition, Nutton (2017a).
156 Eriksson (1959).
157 Garrison (2015).
158 Nutton (2017a: 28). Cornarius had been on friendly terms with Vesalius as recently as the first months of 1543.
159 Below, p. 59; Caius (1544), with the notes in his copy, now Cambridge University Library, classmark Adv, d, 3.1 (formerly Nn.3.19).
160 Below, p. 62.
161 Klestinec (2011); Skaarup (2015).
162 Galen XIX, 13–14 K.; Boudon-Millot (2007: 138).
163 *Anatomy:*Littré (1839–61: 8, 538–40 L): Craik (2006: 119–53).
164 For the techniques of Galen and other earlier commentators on Hippocrates, see Smith (1979); Manetti and Roselli (1994b); Von Staden (2017). Caius, of course, did not know the Galenic commentaries that have survived only in Arabic and were first made available in translation during the twentieth century.
165 For these works, and modern discussions, see Craik (2015: 119–24, 53–6, 224–30 and 166–9 respectively).
166 Caius' achievement would be even more remarkable if he had reached his conclusions before the publication of the great series of Hippocratic commentaries associated with Paris and published from the 1550s onwards. He was more successful in his comments on Galenic tracts, below, pp. 113–81. For Caius as a documentary historian, see Grafton (2017); Nutton (2017b).
167 For developments in anatomy in Italy after Vesalius, see Klestinec (2011); for Cambridge, Jones P (1988a). r
168 Skaarup (2015: 105–11, 127).
169 Alexandrinus (1548); Laguna (1554).
170 Maclean (2002).
171 Galen (1536). The Greek text is entitled *Prognostics from the Time of Taking to one's Bed*, Galen, XIX, 52–28 K. All these texts were quickly dismissed as pseudonymous.
172 Ferretto (2012).
173 For medieval versions, Kudlien and Durling (1991: 117–56).
174 Bylebyl (1991: 173–89).

175 Ongaro (1994) shows conclusively that Da Monte was not the originator of Paduan bedside instruction, and that he had no official standing as a physician employed by the S. Francesco Hospital.

176 Cf. Crato (1563: 348): '*Montanicam prolixitatem nostra breuitate quasi illustremus*'.

177 Caius (1544a).

178 Compare the title of Guinter's (and Vesalius') *Institutiones anatomicae secundum Galenio sententiam, Principles of Anatomy according to the Opinion of Galen*. For the 1544 printing, see Hieronymus (2005: 357, n. 166).

179 Crato's involvement in the religious life of his time has been well studied, from Gillet (1860–61) to Louthan (1994), but his medicine has been badly served. Only a tiny amount of his enormous Europe-wide correspondence was printed in Scholz (1591–1611); more is hinted at in Evans (1973). A full investigation of his medical and natural historical interests is a desideratum.

180 Hieronymus (2005: 1361, n. 388; cf. n. 389–94). In a private letter of 1563 (p. 1382), Crato declares his intention to free Da Monte's ideas from misunderstanding and unjustified reproaches.

181 E.g. Crato (1563: 46: '. . . legant studiosi diuinas Methodos summi Montani'; 396); also in private letters published much later Scholz (1591–1611: I, 200; V, 287–8, complaining of the 'injury' done to him and Da Monte by Donzellini's inclusion of Caius' work); Scholz 1610: 163–6, praise of Da Monte's method; 'what Da Monte would think of some of the books circulating under his name one can only imagine.' [in a letter of 1557].

182 Da Monte (1558). Not discussed in Hieronymus (2005).

183 Clark (1964: 89–104).

184 Forrester and Henry (2005); Nutton (2008a); Agasss and Pennuto (2016).

185 Spach (1597); King (2007); Van Foreest (1589–1609).

186 Maclean (2002).

187 Gessner (1559); Debus (1965: 52–7).

188 Guinter (1571); Hieronymus (2005: 2480–5).

Part II
Translation: *An Autobibliography*

An Autobibliography by John Caius, from Britain, in one book[1]

To Thomas Hatcher[2]

A few years ago, my dear Thomas, that distinguished and unforgettable scholar Conrad Gessner tried to persuade me to compose a short catalogue of all my writings. I did write something in response to his wishes, but it was quite brief and limited because I did not know exactly why he was asking.[3] Now you are making the same request, and not just a request, for in your most recent letter on the subject you make your case so strongly that it amounts almost to compulsion.[4] You put forward so many reasons and you urge your suit with such powerful eloquence that I may appear to gratify you not out of friendship but because of the strength of your case. When I am in London, you importune me; when I am in Cambridge, you do the same; from near or far, you continually jog my memory, with the result that I wonder just what there could be in the book that /1v would appeal to you. Personally speaking, I certainly cannot see what there is in it that you desire so much. Your wish by itself is a sufficiently good reason for wanting to satisfy you, provided there is nothing here to annoy you or others, and even if there were, provided it is not damaging, I think that that can be left to your goodwill and our friendship, when it is such a pleasure and you are also issuing a sort of order. So here is the book you demand. Since I have no copy of the catalogue I wrote for Gessner to give to you, I shall repeat and rework all the earlier material, adding and appending what I have composed since I wrote to Gessner.[5] I shall also add the reasons and occasions for writing, the persons and circumstances involved, and the places where my writings were published. I shall also explain the titles and almost all the arguments of the books that we wrote, translated or edited, and, as I go along, where necessary, we shall mention disputes among anatomists, the death of the most celebrated Conrad Gessner, and the pronunciation of Greek and Latin according to the opinion and custom of the Greeks, Italians and Germans. We are therefore dedicating this treatise on my own books to you, because you too have been a writer and editor.[6] We shall go through everything in chronological order, beginning with my early years.

When I was in my twenty second year and still a student at Cambridge here in Britain, in order to gratify my friends and to test /2r my own abilities, I made some translations from Greek into Latin: as well as some from Latin

Translations.

into the vernacular as seemed appropriate for the instruction of those for whom I wrote them.[7] I translated from Greek into Latin for a friend the little book of the Greek Nicephorus Callistus Xanthopoulus in which he explains how a man may make his confession simply by praying.[8] Likewise, the little book of Chrysostom on praying to God, for a gentleman at court because he did not seem to be much given to prayer.[9] I further produced an abridgement of Erasmus' book on true theology for another person who, although keen to read the holy scriptures, did not know the appropriate boundaries of reading and studying them, or how he might safely discover them.[10] (There was at that time a new form of religion beginning to spread widely in England.)[11] Finally, I translated a *Paraphrase of the Epistle of Jude* for another friend who was keen to study this Epistle.[12] These were my juvenile writings.

Commentaries on the poems of Framingham.

Six years later, there died in Norwich on September 29th, 1537, at the age of 25 years, seven months and six days, our friend William Framingham, a fellow townsman, educated from childhood at the same school in Norwich as us. He was a man possessed of a most tenacious memory, a fertile intelligence, wide reading, and tireless endeavour and diligence. He was educated in his youth at Pembroke Hall, Cambridge, then in early manhood made a Fellow of Queens' College; by calling a philosopher, by degree /2v a Master of Arts though men spoke of him as a Doctor of Arts.[13] A young man of honeyed eloquence, he was deeply acquainted with all the liberal arts (especially music and rhetoric, in which he was outstanding), the poets, historians and theologians (for he was learned in both Greek and Latin).[14] On his death bed, he entrusted to me all the books he had written in his lifetime.

He had written eight in all. He wrote on *Continence* in two books of elegant prose, in which he vigorously attacked brothels and the sex trade to such an extent that he refused even to acknowledge the Poets, those professors of love; he condemned lust, and praised chastity, proposing punishments for one and rewards for the other. His other books he wrote in verse on a variety of themes. He wrote in hexameters and pentameters a single book *A Consolation, for Aemilianus, a Blind Man*, in which he consoled himself for the weak eyesight he had brought on through excessive study in Cambridge, setting out the advantages we obtain through blindness as well as the psychological inconveniences we avoid.[15] There follows a fourth work, *Laurence*, an epic poem on the martyrdom of St Laurence, whose content he summarises in the following lines:

> His hovel torched and burnt to the ground, / the deceits of the crafty Detius, the furious plots of young men, / these are our song; the glory won by our hero, and the shades that enveloped sad Mezentius.[16]/3r

The fifth is *Ecpyrosis*, or the burning of the Sodomites by heavenly fire for their evil crimes, obscene lust and turpitude, also in heroic verse.[17] Sixth, *Idolatry*, in which by using the treasured words of Scripture but even more those of Poetry he denounces in glyconic choriambic verse those who in his own day have left the worship of the true God for that of sad idols.[18] He says that gluttons worship their bellies as gods, drunkards Bacchus; brawlers Mars; the lustful Venus; misers Plutus, listing in turn in this way all pagan and foreign deities, and declaring that the human race adores and worships them as gods when through a multitude of sins it departs and falls away from the true God.

The seventh he called *Arete*, the Greek word for virtue. In it he shows that the strength and power of virtue is all-sufficient for the good life; no adversity can put down virtue from its seat. Virtue is eternal and without end; it is not consumed by fire, or constrained by chains; never dominated by authority or harmed by an enemy; it conserves justice, repels lust, puts drunkenness to flight, drives out other vices, and takes its seat in heaven.

The eighth is a book of *Epigrams*, varied in both theme and metre, in two books, whose argument would be too long to explain.[19] We wrote notes and commentary on all these when we were young, both because they were rather obscure to anyone except the learned because of /3v their stories, their words and phrases from the poets, their descriptions of stars, seasons and regions, their half-lines, allusions and alternative names, as well as the various ways in which were depicted facts, ideas and arguments; and also because it had always given me great pleasure, from my youth onwards, so to speak, to review my proficiency in the classical languages at the time and subsequently in other areas of knowledge.[20] But both commentaries and books disappeared without hope of recovery from among those with whom I had left them when I set out for Italy, although I carefully searched for them on my return and up until the present year of writing, 1570.[21] But last April, when I mentioned the books while at table with the most reverend Matthew [Parker], Archbishop of Canterbury, Edmund [Guest], Bishop of Rochester, who was also there, declared that they survived in his library, and in printed form, as far as his memory went, promising to return them to me as soon as he had time.[22] But since we have not yet received them, we have not been able to publish them.

We also began a history of our home town of Norwich in Eastern Britain, mentioned by the ancient writers Cornelius Tacitus and Antoninus Augustus under the name of Nordovicum and Venta respectively.[23] We intended to finish it, but various pursuits both public and private impeded any progress and prevented completion, although we still have an undigested draft. I should not dare to make any promises about the future, /4r but if the fates allow and we have time, we will perhaps continue with what we have begun, if not to the very end, but at least as far as we are able.[24] Even if not, we will provide a taster in the book which we have written on the ancient towns of Britain.[25] Meanwhile we think it better to say nothing about it than to write only a little.

History of the city of Norwich.

These are our first books. The next we wrote in 1542 when we were still a young student at university in Italy, the two books that we entitled *The Method of Healing according to Galen and Giambattista da Monte*, my

The Method of Healing.

teacher in medicine.[26] In writing them we held close to their line of thought, as did Galen and Celsus to that of Hippocrates, Oribasius and Paul [of Aegina] to that of Galen, and Vergil to that of Homer (as Macrobius clearly shows from a comparison between the two), and indeed there is no-one who does not choose somebody to imitate.[27] Not only did I copy everything down by hand, but also by carefully reasoning about everything I extracted the very pith and marrow of the topics and the language, like shelling a nut, and then provided a version of everything in my own way. By following this plan, we gave the overall sense of his thought, but not in the simple and unstructured words or the disjointed phrases and ideas of his lectures (although they were all extremely learned).[28] We weighed our words rather than merely counting them. An unprejudiced and open-minded reader will very easily discover this by a careful comparison between our *Method* and that of Da Monte (which is now available among his publications /4v but was not so at the time), and by an even more careful assessment of their material, order, style and overall purpose in writing.[29] But if we have watered our tiny plots from the streamlets of others, as Cicero boasts he did, will they not still remain our tiny plots?[30] For otherwise the books that he wrote 'according to the opinion of Hippocrates' will no longer belong to Galen; or the three books on the movement of the lung and thorax which he says contain teaching material from his master Pelops; or that book on medical experience which, on his own admission, he had composed on the basis of the ideas of Pelops and Philip the Empiricist.[31] Indeed, in his own autobibliography he says that Pelops and Philip the Empiricist held a debate in which Pelops took the view that medicine could not be constituted by experience alone, and Philip that it could, and that, after he had heard the views expressed on either side and put them into order, he wrote them up as a sort of private essay.[32] No longer will there belong to Epicurus the books that Marcus Tullius [Cicero] records as having been drawn by Epicurus from the springs of Democritus.[33] Nor will Marcus Cicero have that book about the universe that he took largely from Plato's *Timaeus*, nor the work *On Duties*, for which, in Book II, he admits to having drawn substantially on Panaetius, as well as the many other things that he plucked almost verbatim out of Xenophon.[34] His readers know how much he delights and rejoices that his gardens are abloom with their flowers, as if it were a great achievement.[35] Nor can one forget his proud boast to Atticus that he had used up the whole perfume-cabinet of Isocrates in his writings.[36] Besides, the five books of Theophilus /5r Protospatharius on the make-up of the human body will not belong to Theophilus, since they are only an abridgement of Galen's *The Use of Parts*.[37] Nor will Plautus and Terence be the owners of the comedies that they for the most part translated from Menander and Apollodorus,[38] or Pythagoras of the material which Alexander Polyhistor reports he took from Zoras the Assyrian.[39] Nor is the great Poem Homer's, since Bocchus shows that he inserted into his work many lines from the Delphic Sybil, who prophesied the events of the Trojan War

The Nature of the Gods, Book I.

long before they occurred.[40] Livy is not the author of his Book XXI, which would seem to have been translated almost literally from Polybius.[41] Much of Planudes is really Cato's, and, to come to recent authors, Erasmus' *Apothegms* were assembled out of Plutarch, Athenaeus, Xenophon and others.[42] Need I say more? The *Therapeutic Method* which he says he wrote according to Galen and Da Monte will no longer belong even to Crato.[43] Indeed, one may go so far as to say that no one knows everything, or is so confident of his own resources that he does not need a Theseus; no one is entirely self-sufficient.[44] Even Jupiter called in the Titans to help.[45] Certainly, the anatomical portions that go under the name of Oribasius are even less likely to be his, for they are almost entirely derived verbatim from Galen. Indeed, he did not, like us, copy only the ideas of Galen, but he took over almost everything word for word. He copied everything in the first section from *Anatomical Procedures; /5v* the second contains almost the whole of *Bones*, as well as the whole of Galen's *Anatomy of Muscles and Nerves*.[46] Those who want can find just about everything there. Yet for this reason I am so far from thinking of them as not his (since he specifically admits that his anatomical sections come from Galen) that I consider that he deserves considerable thanks from everyone for preserving for us what time and neglect have otherwise taken from us.[47] This was why I decided to edit the two books on the dissection of muscles and nerves as soon as I had time.[48] Although I shall give great credit to Da Monte, my teacher from whom I learned a great deal, I should not wish for that reason to wrong Galen (his teacher, from whom he derived all the method that he imparted to us, his audience) and myself. For just as more was taken from Galen than from Da Monte, so some things came out of our own workshop (to speak rather modestly about myself). So, if there is anyone in the past, present or future who should take this away from us, we will have justice on our side when we claim that we have been injured for certain; especially because we clearly admitted that what we had written largely derived from their ideas, and we ascribed even our comments to their names. Whoever does not know this should read our two books published in Roman script at Basle in 1544 by Hieronymus Froben and Nicolaus Episcopius.[49] Meanwhile, and incidentally, it is a pleasure to know that our books on the method of healing are seen to be inspired by Galen and Da Monte and that we are not considered to have departed from them for the /6r worse. These two books contain only a general methodology.[50] As far as a specific practice or a particular method of healing is concerned, you may discover this in my two books on *The English Fever*, which will be found to be a singular instance and exemplar of method, should you desire to treat the sick methodically, as indeed you ought.[51] Those who give the title of 'methods' to epitomes and summaries, or brief digests of chapters (like Leonhard Fuchs in the *Letter to Fabritius* prefaced to his book that he rightly called a compendium of medicine, but in no way correctly a method) do not seem to me to understand what method is, begging their pardon.[52]

Galen's anatomy of muscles and nerves.

At the same time, we wrote commentaries on the nine extant books of Galen's *Anatomical Procedures* and the two of *The Movement of Muscles*, which we collated with similar attention in Italy against an old book that the very famous Lazzaro Bonamico, then public professor of Greek and Latin humane letters at Padua, allowed me to use.[53] In addition, in editing the former, some notes, but pretty few, were taken from an old Greek book in the possession of the Giuntas, thanks to Agostino Gadaldino, assuredly a very helpful and learned man, who was then head of the Giuntine Press.[54] They had been passed on to Andreas Vesalius for use in editing Latin translations of Galen's anatomical writings. He was then sharing a house for eight months with me in Padua i.e. Casa degli Valli or, as the Paduans say, Ca' Valle, near the Ponte della /6v Paglia, while he was writing and illustrating his books on the *Fabric of the Human Body*.[55] Antonio Giunta, Agostino Ricci and Vettore Trincavelli were at the time engaged in an honourable rivalry to produce a more accurate edition of the complete works of Galen in Latin.[56] But these notes proved of little value to me and Vesalius (for they were for the most part unreliable), although they did provide an opportunity to look more closely for other copies.[57] In my researches I found another Greek copy owned by Bessarion in the Library of St Mark's in Venice, which helped in some

places.[58] Having edited the nine surviving books on anatomy by Galen and prepared a commentary on them, on my way back to England I arranged for them to be published at Basle by Hieronymus Froben and Nicolaus Episcopius in 1544, together with the complete text of Galen's *Substitute Drugs*, most of which had been adopted by Paul of Aegina for his own purposes; most of book VII of Galen's *The Use of Parts* in Greek; the first book of Galen's *The Opinions of Hippocrates and Plato* in Greek, together with my Latin translation; Galen's book on *Coma;* and the Greek text of Hippocrates, *Drugs*, which had not previously been found and published.[59] At the end of *Drugs* there was a substantial section which Paulo Grassi, one of my medical professors, made into a fifth chapter.[60] But because it/ 7r was entirely irrelevant here and was taken word for word from Hippocrates' *The Art of Medicine*, I believe by a scholar who had lumped many things together in a single manuscript, we deliberately ignored it and decided to exclude it completely; anyone who is interested may find it in its proper place.[61] When I returned to Britain, I obtained another copy of *Anatomical Procedures*, belonging to the

Englishman John Clement, an upright man and a remarkable doctor, and another owned by Thomas Linacre, a man of excellent judgment, who, among his many great achievements, founded the London College of Physicians in 1520. (We wrote its *Annals* from the foundation of the College until 1565, the last year of our Presidency.)[62] We were President for seven years, as far as the building of our College in Cambridge allowed: it was begun in 1565 and finished in 1570.[63] We also wrote the *Annals of Gonville College, Cambridge*, from its beginnings until the present year, 1570; you may read its general argument in our *History of Cambridge University*.[64] These histories were written merely for the private use of both Colleges, whereas the copies of Linacre and Clement we obtained were for public use. We added much from them to what we had already edited in preparation for a second edition I have planned to go with my own Greek edition of Galen's *The Use of Parts*.[65] We were particularly keen on this because that particular work of Galen is in my view necessary and valuable for men of all kinds.[66] Physicians and surgeons by learning from /7v it about the human condition can thereby discover how to use, respectively, drugs and the knife, as we explained in Book II of my *Method of Healing*.[67] Philosophers with an interest in the natural world may learn to admire the nature of humankind and the miracle of Nature in it. But everyone may use it to find out about themselves, for there is nothing more pleasing to contemplate than this.[68] For who will not know himself better when he understands what parts he has, and how they are fitted and joined together? I am only extremely sorry that the remaining books of Galen's treatise have never been seen by anyone, as far as I know, for many years.[69] Ambrosio Calepino under the rubric '*medicina*' in the edition of Hagenau, 1526, declares that a great part of this anatomical treatise was once in the possession of one Antonio Visconti (I think in Italy).[70] We also added commentaries on the same tract, where, among other things, we spoke about the hinge joint which modern anatomists have depicted wrongly; about the septum in the brain that does not act as a support but as a divider, which is discussed in a passage in *Anatomical Procedures*, Book IX, badly emended by Vesalius; and about the deltoid muscle and tying a knot, in order to make these passages intelligible.[71] We have also stated that there are not ten abdominal muscles (as is believed by those who only count muscles from their outlines, and include as two the two tiny appendages at the lower end of the straight muscles). We accept only eight along with Galen and those who number them /8r according to their function and purpose.[72] There are just two straight muscles (about which there is the argument). We merely provided a summary then, without giving reasons. We shall repeat them here, relying on the fundamentals established by Galen. We agree with Galen that every muscle takes its origin from a bone and is inserted into a bone. That is so because it draws and moves bones, the chief instruments and bases of the body. The fleshy mass is not provided in order to be moved (that happens incidentally through the movement of the bone to which it is attached), but so that it may be an instrument of motion and move the limbs, like puppet strings.[73] The bone is passive, whereas the fleshy mass is active, hence it takes its appellation 'muscle' from *motus*, i.e. *movisculum* 'little mover'. If I am not mistaken it takes its name 'mys' from the outline of a mouse [in Greek μῦς], which it very greatly resembles, if you remove its skin and paws.[74] It cannot draw or move anything if it is not firmly attached to something at each end, i.e. that towards which the attraction takes place and that which is drawn; the former provides it with stability, the latter something to clasp and hold. The drawing motion in the limbs is rather like men hauling together on a rope to move

Only eight abdominal muscles.

something or themselves in a tug of war, one pulling, the other resisting. In both cases it is essential that the rope is either tied round or is very firmly held by each side. When this is done and they pull vigorously, with men the stronger drags the weaker wherever he wants, or the object that is pulled follows with difficulty if it is heavy, easily if it is light. Pulling cannot happen in any other way. Now if in order to produce movement the muscle must be fixed firmly at each end, i.e. at its points of origin and insertion, to a bone (I do not mean to just one, but to another as well)/8v as the old anatomists taught, then those little fleshy straps will not be muscles because they are not inserted into a bone.[75] So it rightly follows that there are only two straight muscles, because each of the straight muscles is firmly fixed at one end to the breast bone, at the other to the pubic bone. Hence it follows that if there were four straight muscles, there would also be four different bones to which they were attached. Since this is not so (for there is no bone between the xiphoid process and the pubic bone but only the abdomen), it cannot be true that there are four straight muscles, but only two, one on each side. But if you were to claim that what they call tiny muscles in producing movement have the job of the tail ends which are spliced into the main rope in ringing a heavy bell, i.e. as subsidiary tools for movement, I would reject that too, because at their ends they are not affixed by firm sinews but by weak processes, and not to rigid bones on each side, but to wobbly flesh.[76] Not forgetting that they do not move (if they were to move) in the same way as the straight [muscles] but in the opposite way, for the movement and drawing motion of the straight muscles is not downwards, but upwards, with their heads placed in the chest, whereas that of the flaps is the reverse. That said, it is an axiom of anatomy that each one pulls towards its origin, unless to defend your case, you are forced to argue that the straight muscles have their origin in the pubic bone, not the breast bone. But that is something that has been rejected until now by all /9r the older anatomists, who have been extremely skilled in dissecting the human body.[77] Otherwise there is no reason why you should wish to place their heads in the pubic bone, except perhaps for the chest to be moved downwards. But the chest does this by its own weight when the countervailing muscles relax, without any muscles pulling it down. Indeed, to raise the lower parts of the body, which with their own weight resist being moved upwards, needs muscular force to an enormous degree.[78] That is why their heads are situated at the top. But although the pelvis does not have the same natural movement as a joint, it is moved by the motion of something else, that of the spine, as can be easily seen in sexual activity and similar movements. If the pubic bone were not moved, consequently the muscle head would not be placed there and the tendon in the breastbone for that movement. It could be said likewise that the breastbone is not moved, since the roots of the ribs are firmly tied to the transverse processes of the vertebrae in such a way that none can be naturally moved individually. But they all can do so together as a consequence of the flexing of the spine, their own weight and that of the upper parts, and the

Margin notes:

Fleshy straps at the root of the straight [muscles] are not muscles.

Straight [muscles] do not have their origin in the pubic bone.

relaxation of the muscles that stretch and extend it. Nor will you locate the heads of the muscles at the bottom unless you are going against the natural order and the dictate of reason, for all the muscles which go downwards in a straight line take their origin from upper areas. To begin at the top, those moving the jaw have the origin in the skull, those the upper arm in the shoulder, those the ulna in the upper arm, those the hand in the ulna. Those that move the upper legs originate in the hips (/9v), those that move the tibias in the upper leg, those that move the feet in the tibias. There is a good reason for that, for, since all upwards movement is vigorous through having to counteract the weight of the parts below, it needs the assistance of muscles to produce movement. On the other hand, the weight of each part is enough in itself for downwards movements (unless deliberately blocked by opposing muscles), except when there is some particular requirement for vigorous action. Even if the flaps have oblique fibres, they would not be muscles simply by virtue of that fact (for there is flesh with transverse fibres between the radius and ulna down to the wrist, which, nevertheless, is not a muscle); but even if they were muscles, they would only move with an oblique motion, for obliqueness cannot provoke anything other than an oblique movement, were movement to occur at all. However, I do not think that they do provide movement, but in my view they simply cushion and fill up [space] (like the flesh that I have said is placed between the radius and ulna down to the wrist) and provide protection.[79] Indeed, there is a tendon going from the straight muscle underneath which would be damaged by being squashed, if the flesh around it did not prevent an injury by acting as a sort of cushion. But why should I seriously pursue these fancies that Galen scarcely deigned to mention? Why should I talk about the insertions in the straight muscles or explicate their function, when it seemed good to Galen to pass them and similar trivia over in silence, and concentrate only on essentials? You can tell this from his comment at the end of his introductory book on bones, where he says that he will deliberately say nothing about the bone in the heart, larynx or nose, the sesamoid and other similar minor ones, until he has described everything that is essential to know.[80] He adds his reason: they do not need to be described at this point, /10r explaining that he intended to put down and pursue only the essentials, and to omit everything trivial and unimportant. Indeed, Galen's argument can be justified and free him from any imputation of ignorance or negligence. If those who criticise Galen so much knew this, they would stop their aspersions. If they had to discover everything that he discovered and establish all the fundamentals that he did without a Theseus to guide them, they all would be fairer and more charitable to Galen, and they would not attack him so viciously and unfairly with a sharp pen and a biting tongue.[81] But since he left out only a few minor things, and modern authors have received all the essential knowledge they have from Galen alone, and have rendered it their own by rewriting it in a different style and order, and, besides, since they have pointed to just a few trivia (so to speak) that Galen had either

The insertions in the straight [muscles].

neglected or thought little of, or that they have added as a result of an incompetent dissection, it is remarkable what novelties they claim to have discovered, and how great the song and dance they make against Galen, as if it were a matter of house and home, and everything came out of their own workshop.[82] Yet they scarcely agree among themselves, and fail to explain functions, but only teach mostly what is not there.[83] I praise diligence, when it does not damage or pull down a great man, the like of whom the world has not seen since his death and medicine will not see in the future. An earlier century came close to worshipping him, as Eusebius testifies,/10v and we should embrace him with both arms for the monumental writings we have received.[84] We will then see that we are by far his inferiors, if we consider everything with an open mind and without pandering to prejudice. But youth is a bitter thing, and bitter also temerity and self-love.[85] I shall, however, mention briefly the insertions; they were not formed by nature according to the number of straight muscles but to provide strength and stability. For if Nature had divided them by number, she would have fixed one into the bone at each point of origin and insertion, whereby, as has been said earlier, they could individually provide assistance when the bone had to be moved. But since there is only one point of origin and one insertion in a straight muscle, more insertions do not make more muscles (for not every division makes a muscle), but they make it more stable. For because of the sinewy interlacings, [tendinous intersections] the fleshy parts (soft and weak as they are) become shorter and easily make up for any weakness in the length. For several short portions [of a muscle] are more tenacious and less liable to damage than a single long one, just as a short rope is tougher and stronger than a long one. In addition, the intersections make for a more effective and elegant motion of the limb in movement. If the muscle were continuous without any intersection, like that in the femur of a runner, through its roles in movement the belly would swell excessively and inelegantly and would be in danger of rupture, something that Nature always avoids./82 For its size hampers performance, its appearance offends the eye; and there is always a risk of harm in straining,/11r as Galen writes in his treatise on anatomy once happened to the muscle of a runner.[86] But if the muscles are divided and separated into more and shorter parts, they swell only moderately, since the major role of a single one is distributed among the lesser roles of several. In that way, both its duty is well served and elegance satisfied. We also warned the reader in these commentaries or notes of some places in the anatomy books that Vesalius had corrupted after Antonio Giunta, the Venetian printer, had entrusted him with the task of editing them.[87] Among them is *Anatomical Procedures*, Book 9, p. 335, on the septum in the brain.[88] We also added, p. 299, a true picture of the *ginglymus* in accordance with Galen's opinion, which is very different from and clearly unlike what Vesalius earlier expressed in the first edition of his book in 1543, p. 14, where his description does not allow a join from both sides as in the *ginglymus* joint in the bones of the human body[89] (Figure 7).

Function of the insertions.

Editions.

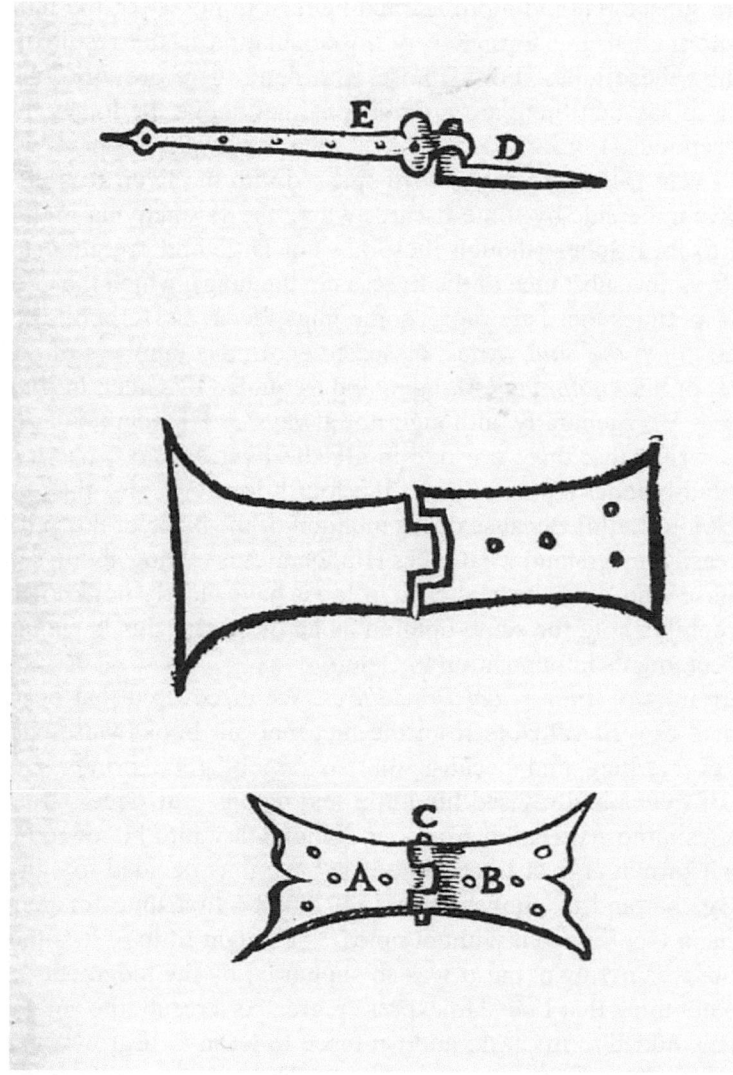

Figure 7 The *ginglymus* hinge as depicted by Vesalius and Caius: top: Vesalius, *Fabrica* 1543: p. 14: middle: Caius, *Libri aliquot* 1544: 299: bottom Vesalius, *Fabrica*, ed. 2, 1555: p. 17.

    In the same commentary we said a few words about the lobes in the liver, which the Greeks call λόβοι, because there was a debate both then and now with Galen on the number of the lobes.[90] Modern writers suggest that there are either none or two, the ancients declare that there are two, three or more, the greater or lesser number depending on whether the liver is big or small.[91]

The more substantial and more learned believe in the latter, the lightweight and uninformed in the former. Any miscalculation is the result of misunderstanding these lobes. For if those who deny there are any lobes at all are going to say that there are no divisions that define the lobes, they deny their perceptions,/11v for the liver is divided into two main parts where the umbilical vein [*inferior vena cava*] is passed into the liver. It is divided on its concave underside by some fissures where the parenchyma in the middle rises up to form lobes (though these are not large and are almost entirely distinct from the substance of the liver, as in the lung), which the Greeks call λόβοι. Sometimes these are more, sometimes fewer, as Herophilus (who, as Tertullian in *On the Soul* writes, dissected enormous numbers of men) says in book II of his *Anatomical Matters*, and as quoted by Galen in *Anatomical Procedures* VI, 'generally, although not always'.[92] Hippocrates in his book *Anatomy* writes that there are five in all: the liver, he says, has five lobes, and the gall-bladder rests on top of the fourth lobe.[93] [Caius then translates the Greek into Latin] Because of his mention of the place of the gall-bladder one can easily understand what lobes Hippocrates is talking about, something which those who deny the existence of lobes have clearly not known. Galen and Herophilus hold the same opinion as he did.[94] But this is enough about fanciful comments in opposition to Galen.

I return now to *Anatomical Procedures*. We discovered that our work in editing had proved valuable from the fact that our books were widely circulated everywhere and because that extremely good printer Guillaume Rouille of Lyons had revised his Latin text against our Greek, transferring many notes almost verbatim from our commentary into his own, published in a small format /12r at Lyons in 1551.[95] We thus decided to edit Galen's book *Hygiene*, and to publish it in 1549 for the first time for general use with Johann Oporinus but without notes.[96] I thought little of it, although the endeavour was my own, but it was so supported by the judgments of others that I do not think that I need to express regret. As a result, the enthusiasm of others only added to my task, and I refused to let myself grow weary when I saw others so eager for me to carry it out. The spur to editing *Hygiene* was as follows. The Englishman Henry Knolles, a very kind and extremely close friend, when we were together in Padua, easily persuaded me as a mark of our friendship to read with him Galen's *Hygiene* in Greek.[97] I employed the utmost care possible in providing him with an improved text. In order to fix what he had heard more firmly in his memory, as he was a generous man, he used to repeat at midday in front of Italians whatever I used to expound with him in the morning, assuredly to great universal thanks. Although I had satisfied him as a man devoted to the Classics, I had not, however, satisfied myself as a student of medicine. For everything was full of mistakes. So having got hold of several copies in Italy and also on my return in England (two of which were provided to me by the celebrated physicians John Clement

Commentaries on Galen's Hygiene.

H. Knolles.

and George Owen),/12v we wanted to produce a text carefully corrected as far as possible.[98] Because I understood that my earlier commentaries on other books had gained favour and been useful (for I observed that many have spent time in reading them), I did not refrain from providing notes on this text also; for they were necessary because of changes in wording and in *Realien*, as well as to give advice to careful readers.[99] Later I handed over the finished books and the accompanying commentary to the printer Johann Oporinus in Basle to be printed in 1563, adding Galen's books *To Thrasybulus* and *The Small Ball* in Greek, also edited by me, since they seemed to relate to the same theme. We also added annotations to each book, because some things required illustration, some advice to the reader, and some explanation. We also added a book by Galen in Greek, *Humours*, which I had emended in several places.[100] We prefixed a letter to Lady Anne, wife of Sir Nicholas Bacon, Keeper of the Great Seal of England, a woman most learned in Greek and Latin and a member of the most educated Cooke family, all of whose members, both male and female, can today be compared with that most famous family of Thomas More in the past.[101] Since we have mentioned them, we cannot also fail to record the very great learning of our late queen Mary and our present queen Elizabeth, Mildred, wife of esteemed Cecil, Margaret, wife of John Clement, and Margaret,/13r wife of William Roper, and other notable women we remember as well as others earlier in Britain.[102] In addition to the books just mentioned, Oporinus undertook to publish something long desired by many people as well as him, the commentary by the most learned John Claymond on the complete *Natural History* of Caius Pliny, especially the first two books, which had disappeared on his death but which I had requested from the President of Corpus Christi College, Oxford (over which Claymond presided in his lifetime) to please Johann Oporinus, who had importuned me in many letters.[103] But I am not sufficiently aware of why he postponed this edition. For he has not yet printed my books or those of Claymond, although in the case of the latter I had asked him several times to return them to me, not just in my letters, but through my friends, including the excellent Sir Christopher Mounte, Doctor of Laws, and for a long time a distinguished representative of the rulers of England in Strasbourg, and John Gylpin, a very kind man.[104] But whether through a lack of funds or because of that human failing to long for what you have not got, but to despise it once you have it, I know not.[105] And I would now be afraid of my books becoming an object of dispute, now he is dead, were I not well aware that the executors of his will are men of learning and probity. I strongly beg them either to publish the books or to return them safe to me.[106]

We also edited a few other books by Galen, such as the complete text of *The Opinions of Hippocrates and Plato*;/13v whose first book we discovered by chance; all of *The Method of Healing* and all of *The Properties of Simple Drugs*; and all the books that Galen entitled *The Composition of Drugs*, in

(margin notes: John Clement, G. Owen. / *Thrasybulus, The Small Ball* / Galen's *Humours*. / Learned ladies. / John Claymond's books with Oporinus. / Christopher Mounte. / Editions.)

Wrong titles.

17 books.[107] Some divide these last into *The Composition of Drugs, by Site* and *The Composition of Drugs by Type*, and give them separate numbers, as if they were distinct guides to compounding remedies, and not a single comprehensive work, or, as Galen termed it, a 'treatise'. In this they clearly make the same error as when they divide into two the single book on *The Stages of Illness*, when what they make into a separate part II is simply part of Book I, where he is dealing first with specific stages of disease, and then with them in general.[108] That is why one should entitle the whole book *The Stages of Illness*, and make it clear in a marginal note where Galen begins to talk about stages of disease in general. I think that this is what a scholar first did, but then a scribbler made a title out of the note. I am surprised that translators have not noticed this in both treatises, or realised that the book on the compounding of drugs was not split between several books and titles, putting *Drugs, by Site* before *By Type*./14r That *By Type* comes first, and *By Site* follows in such a way that the last book of *By Type* is Book VII of *The Compounding of Drugs*, and the first of *By Site* Book VIII of *The Compounding of Drugs*, and so on. We also corrected Galen's books *Affected Parts*, adding summaries of each book, *The Differences between Fevers, The Power of Purgatives*, as well as the little book in which Galen explains who should be purged, how and

Wrong book numbers.

when. We also prepared a better text of *The Differences between Diseases*; likewise, the single book of *The Causes of Disease*, the single book of *The Differences between Symptoms*; and the three books of *The Causes of Symptoms*. All these were first printed in Greek at Basle together as six books of the same work; with the book *The Differences between Diseases* coming first, *The Causes of Disease* second, *The Differences between Symptoms* third; *The Causes of Symptoms*, Book I fourth, Book II fifth, and Book III sixth, really quite wrongly and very far from what Galen had devised.[109] We will say more of this in the book that we wrote in Greek about the books of Galen that are no longer extant, where we will also show the order of his works.[110] But this is enough about the Greek books of Galen that were emended. There follow /14v the books in Latin that were edited by me.

Celsus.

In 1543 when I finished my job of lecturing on the teachings of Aristotle in Greek with a public salary from the illustrious Venetians, I planned a trip around Italy before my return to Britain.[111] (I taught at the same hour as Realdo Colombo of Cremona, in the general schools by S. Biagio in Padua, for the schools of the Artists were still in the course of construction at the Bo' [Figure 8] and were not separate from the schools of the jurists.)[112] So in July of that year I left Padua for Florence and Pisa to hear that celebrated scholar Matteo Corti, our teacher in medicine.[113] I carried with me a copy of Celsus on my journey, having copied three manuscripts in Florence at the public library of the most illustrious Cosmo de' Medici at San Lorenzo, which thanks to the kindness and generosity of the prince is open to all students of literature, and I devoted careful attention to removing through my studies the harm done to Celsus.[114] I was certainly sorry for the damage he suffered through the ravages

M. Corti.

The library at Florence.

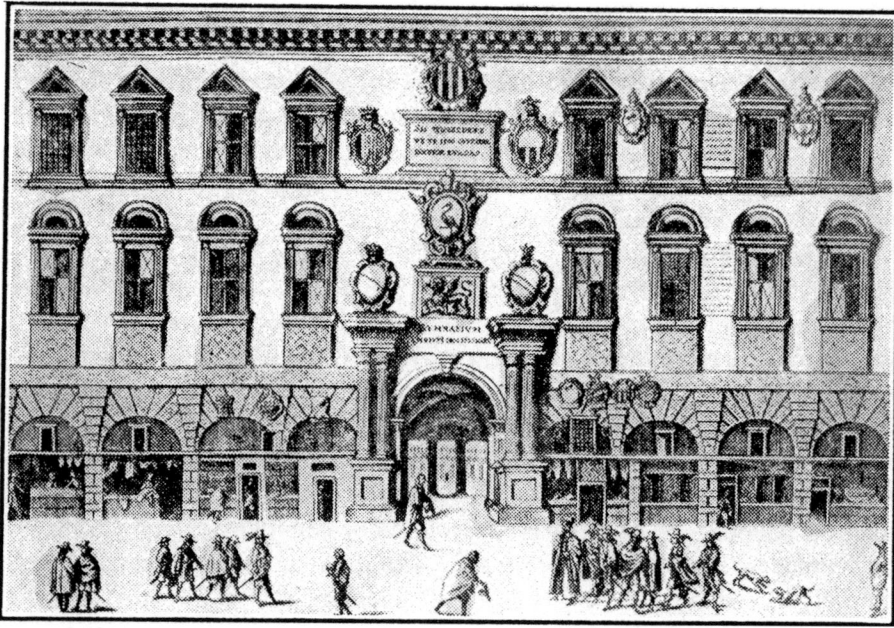

Figure 8 The Bo' at Padua, built while Caius was teaching there.

Copyright Wellcome Collection.

of time and men. I bemoaned the fact that the eloquence of a great man, who should be rightly considered the chief among Latin doctors, should be so corrupted and his medicine lie neglected. When I decided to render assistance to him, I collated with the three Florentine codices (one very old, the others more recent) the Celsus printing, Lyons, 1542, which seemed to me to be a better text. I also compared it with the editions of Venice /15r and Solingen.[115] When I had my doubts about these, I consulted another manuscript from Urbino, which we managed to see in the library of the Duke of Urbino only after three days of entreaties (along with the books of Galen, *The Use of Parts, Hippocrates' Aphorisms* and *the Introduction or the Doctor*).[116] Whether access to the Library is so difficult because he is like that in mind and nature or because a little earlier he had been rudely treated by a printer to whom he had loaned the complete book of Galen's *Drugs Easy to Hand*, or for some other reason, I know not.[117] On our return to Padua we also had access to another manuscript copy, owned by Lazzaro Bonamico, an extremely eloquent speaker at Padua.[118] If these were not enough, for quite often one leaned one way, another another, we also consulted Hippocrates himself, because Celsus imitates him just as Marcellus does Scribonius, Vergil Homer, and Oribasius Galen, but so invisibly that you can only grasp this if you are well versed in Hippocrates.[119] When I returned to Britain I collated others when I had time, and revised everything I had transcribed in Italy. By this means we were freed from the various scruples from which

The library at Urbino.

Celsus interpreter of Hippocrates.

many outstanding scholars, once entrapped, cannot yet disentangle themselves and from a variety of doubts. We made several emendations to passages that had been investigated by many but resolved by none (to judge from their writings). Where codices differed or were silent because of some corruption and /15v we could not obtain what we most wanted for the reasons already mentioned, we were forced to employ our considered judgment, but in such a way that we advised the reader in a short note that if our comment did not quite fit, he would be free to make his own judgment or follow that of someone else as he thought right. The treatises were very often at odds with one another, especially those copied recently, because they have often been corrupted by copyists through being written and rewritten. The old codex, roughly nine hundred years old, had the greater integrity. Of the more recent ones, one belonged to Pietro de' Medici and was written by the elder Antonio di Mario in 1427.[120] The second belonged to Angelo Poliziano, a most polished scholar, whose ownership I established from his personal subscription, and was copied by the younger Antonio di Mario in 1453. Before our commentaries on Celsus and Scribonius we inserted a preface dealing with the style and argument of Celsus, the weights and measures used by Celsus and Scribonius, and the true character and design of the Roman denarius, which we had drawn and engraved after the design of a silver Roman denarius we own. We also added an extremely full index of all significant topics.[121]

Ancient copies of Celsus.

Scribonius.

Having finished with Celsus, it came into my mind to edit Scribonius also, an ancient doctor and author, and to compare him with Celsus, because his text was very corrupt and both seemed to be writers in Rome as well as contemporaries./16r Celsus lived in the reign of Tiberius, Scribonius under him, Caligula and Claudius Caesar, whose physician he was and with whom he sailed to Britain, setting sail from the port of Luna (which is the first town in Etruria and still keeps its ancient name).[122] I do not know whether Scribonius wrote his book while in Britain, because he says in one of his recipes that he was abroad and had not access to large numbers of books.[123] We edited Scribonius largely, although not entirely, by comparing Marcellus, who took a great deal verbatim from Scribonius (as Paul, Aetius and Oribasius did from Galen), and repeated it with variant wording, as well as leaving much out, namely, what Largus had written about plasters, poisons and antidotes, and epilepsy. Whenever we had to introduce our own judgment either if Marcellus was missing or the text itself was corrupt, we supplied a brief commentary, just as we have explained above.[124] I still have my Celsus and Scribonius edited, put together, and provided with notes, and will publish them as soon as my free time allows. Meanwhile fortune has decreed that these which were edited first should be handed to the printers after *Hygiene*, which was edited later.[125]

The British Fever.

After finishing them, there began in 1551 an outbreak in England of our insular plague, which we call the Ephemeral Fever or, by another name, the British Sweat.[126] Because it was at that time/ 16v raging furiously, at the request of Robert Warmington, an especially learned philosopher and London lawyer, as well as in response to the demands of other friends, we first wrote a single book *The British Sweat* for the British public, published by the printer Richard Grafton in London.[127] Because of the rapid spread of the disease it was tossed off in haste rather than carefully composed over time; and then a second version, more accurate, was produced for general benefit.[128] The first was in one book, but then, because of the amount of new material, it was divided into two; in part I we explained at length the causes of the disease and the prophylaxis, in the second its remedies. This book can serve as a good example for students of medicine of the universal method we explained earlier when we made mention of our books on the *Method of Healing*. We were going to link with them three Latin translations of Galen after we had edited them in Greek. Two are Galen's *My own Books* and *The Order of my Books* and the third *Hippocrates' Rationale for Diet in Acute Diseases*.[129] By this I do not mean the commentary he wrote on the Hippocratic tract with that title, but a second little tract, never previously published, which he mentioned in his autobibliography among his writings on therapeutics. I certainly would not have published it yet, because I was not entirely satisfied with the unique Greek copy I used, although I sweated profusely in editing it.[130] (I had felt similarly about the book /17r on *Coma*, which I published for the first time, with others, twenty-five years ago in Basle, except that/I did not want students of medicine to be without the part substantially emended, even if there was still the possibility that it could be published again in a more complete form.)[131] But since I am afraid that, were I to die in the interim, the book would also perish, I shall shortly produce a Greek edition. I decided to make a translation of the other two books rather than an edition, both because I should not like to plunge my sickle into another's harvest, and because it was far easier to make a new translation than to refashion the old or stitch in new and attach new handles to old jugs, since there were so many variations in different places between the earlier widely available Greek exemplars.[132] We will explain our reasoning when we publish our notes on the Greek texts (which, as I said, we have restored) and print them together.[133] These [translations] were printed in italic script at Louvain in 1556 by Antonio Maria Bergagne, an Italian, under the not unfavourable auspices of those who used them in their Latin editions of the complete works of Galen, the latest at Venice in 1565, as will become easily clear to anyone who compares them carefully.[134] We also added an enlarged version of our two books on *The Method of Healing*, providing them with a very full index of topics.

After these had been published, we edited Galen's book in Greek *On Seven-month Children*, and *Characteristics of Hippocrates* /17v (from John of Stobi), which we dedicated to Thomas Wendy, and *Bones for Beginners* (later provided with a short commentary, but not yet published), which we corrected for Thomas Maro.[135] He was passionate about anatomy and a perpetual admirer of Nature. Like Boethus who attended the anatomical

R. Warmington.

Translations.

Galen's *Diet in Acute Diseases*.

Galen's book on *Coma*.

Notes.

Some editions of Galen's works.

dissections of Galen in Rome, for almost twenty years he was a regular attender at the anatomical dissections which we gave for surgeons in London at the instigation of that illustrious prince Henry, the eighth king of that name. (There were none at that time for physicians).[136] [Dr Wendy] would have been very much interested in studies of seven-month births, since Galen's book on that theme had not been edited.[137] We also removed all the chapter divisions from the book on bones, because in the oldest copies we never saw Galen's text divided into chapters; and because, as we recommended in our commentary on Book II of *Anatomical Procedures*, we would always like Galen to be seen as entirely consistent, as, indeed, he is.[138] But we wanted the headings to remain, because we often saw them in very old codices. That they were placed here by Galen (as in *The Properties of Simples, The Properties of Foodstuffs, The Composition of Drugs*, and in many other books) we conjectured from the fact that the first words of Galen that were written after the heading 'On the sacrum', can refer only to the preceding heading.[139] However, one may have doubts about this, since the last heading in the whole book seems to interrupt Galen's wording,/18r which otherwise Galen seems to have written as a continuum, when he says: After these four the ankle ends and the so-called foot begins.[140] The little tract *Barley Gruel* we not only checked against a very old manuscript, but also made it whole, since it had earlier been damaged by a lamp when the then boss of the Aldine press nodded off. Our informant was the Englishman John Clement, an unimpeachable source, a truly outstanding doctor and an acknowledged master of Greek and Latin, who was then at the Aldine Press in Venice. While [the printer] was dozing, a candle fell onto his exemplar and burnt it. These [editions of mine] were printed in Basle in 1557 by Johann Oporinus.[141]

Since then we have edited the Greek text of Hippocrates, *Anatomy*, widely scattered (so we think), but now restored (thanks to our conjecture). Since this book is now far different from what it has been [until now], it is not irrelevant here to add the reasoning behind its restoration. Earlier, when I was going to edit Book VI of Galen's *The Opinions of Hippocrates and, Plato* as well as others, I read there that Galen says he has made an observation on a passage in Hippocrates' *Anatomy of Veins* in Book 2 of his own work on Hippocrates' *Anatomy*.[142] I racked my brains in frustration at this reference, wondering if it was an interpolation or a corruption, and decided to look at Hippocrates' /18v *Anatomy*.[143] Since it was extremely short, no more than twenty lines long, and I found nothing there that I was looking for, I concluded either that the work had suffered considerable damage or, my hypothesis, the books that followed (which I knew related to anatomy) had once been part of Hippocrates' *Anatomy*. Keen to find the actual citation, I read carefully through the tract on *The Heart* and then that on *Glands*, but failed to find what I was seeking.[144] There remained another book, also on anatomy, but because it was entitled *The Nature of Bones*, I thought that my hunt in it for veins would be fruitless. Nevertheless, I took the decision

Galen did not divide his books into chapters.

Barley Gruel.

Hippocrates' *Anatomy.*

to go through it thoroughly. But when I had gone only five lines, the book departed from what its title *The Nature of Bones* had promised in order to deal with the ureters, larynx, lungs, nerves and veins. So, although I found the organisation chaotic and the text corrupt, there dawned a ray of hope of finding what I sought. Thus, proceeding carefully, I came across a passage from Polybus, Hippocrates' pupil, on four pairs of veins, which is utterly untrue and condemned by Galen in his commentary on Hippocrates' *The Nature of Man*, but described by Aristotle in Book III of his *Investigation into Animals* as coming from Syennesis, a Cypriot doctor, and Polybius (one should write 'Polybus').[145] [Aristotle] himself did not adopt the theory, but rejected it. After reading this, there soon followed what I was looking for, namely the anatomy of the veins /19r described in almost the same words as in the section on veins written by Hippocrates in *Epidemics*, Book II, and approved by Galen as Hippocrates' in his commentary on Hippocrates' *The Nature of Man*, Book II, except that it is more complete and two or three lines longer than what is in the *Epidemics*.[146] Once I had found the passage in *The Nature of Man*, I began to realise that all these books, in as much as they were anatomical, ought all to go under the one title of Hippocrates' *Anatomy*, and all under one rubric, although they dealt, under different headings, with different parts of animals. They should not be kept apart under different titles, as before, but copied all together in a single treatise under the title of *Anatomy*. There seemed nothing to prevent this being done, since, as far as I know, nowhere had I read in Hippocrates or Galen that this tract *Anatomy* had been divided up into several individual ones; and, I recalled, nowhere had mention been made by Hippocrates or Galen of the books *The Heart, Glands*, and *The Nature of Bones* under those titles. I also quite often read in Galen's *My own Books* and elsewhere that there were six books of commentary by Galen on this single book of Hippocrates' *Anatomy*.[147] In Book VI of *The Opinions of Hippocrates and Plato* he mentions book II /19v [of his commentary] on *Anatomy*; Book V in *The Seed* Book I; Book III in *Anatomical Procedures* and *Medical Statements in Plato's Timaeus*; and the others elsewhere.[148] He would not have written 'six books' if Hippocrates had composed his *Anatomy* in no more than twenty lines, even if he was rather more expansive in his wording. For that reason, I put the books together, removed their titles and inserted that of *Anatomy*. I paid attention to ensuring that the book should appear better edited, since it had been previously damaged and corrupt in many places, and I made certain that the sections which Calvi indicated had been excised should be replaced.[149] Thus I took the beginning of the book *The Nature of Bones* from the opening of *Leverage*.[150] Since this in Calvi agrees with the beginning of *The Nature of Bones*, it fits here nicely. I also took out whatever seemed to us inauthentic, repetitive or scarcely true. So, we removed the section on the nails, because they are not bones in Galen or Aristotle; and the vertebrae, because of repetition; and we excluded as inauthentic what had been copied from Polybus and Syennesis. I have nothing to say for certain about the order of the books, since they are not put together either in Greek or in the translations by Cornarius, and they were placed in no particular order by Calvi.[151] The tract *Glands*, which he puts first, is separated by many tracts from the others. After these have been put in the right order, there follow/20r the book on *Anatomy* and the book on *The Heart*. Then, after the insertion of Hippocrates' *The Surgery*, comes *The Nature of Bones*. But whether this (which has never been observed as such) or another arrangement was Hippocrates' own cannot be known unless from a complete and accurate copy of Hippocrates' *Anatomy* or from Galen's commentary on it. Now when the truth is so complex, my supposition about the order of the books is that the book long entitled *Anatomy* is the first part which gave its name to the whole. In second place should be *The Nature of Bones* because Galen stated in *The Opinions of Hippocrates and Plato*, Book VI, that he had written on Hippocrates' section on veins (which is in this part) in his Book II. If this part were placed last, as in the printed copies, it is more likely that Galen would have spoken about this in his last books, i.e. V and VI, than in the second. In third place should be the part of *The Heart* which follows neatly on everything that Hippocrates explained about the heart, veins and arteries in *The Nature of Bones*. The latter is not an entire book about bones as is implied by its title (which some copyist seems to have added, as he did with the titles for other books, with little thought for what was being considered in the book as a whole, but only in each part), but just opens with such an account. Finally the last place is claimed for its own by a fourth text,/20v *Glands* (which is linked to *The Heart* by a transition). I give this transition here: 'Let enough be said about the heart; this now deals with the general nature of glands.'

Layout of the books of Hippocrates' Anatomy.

I decided to publish them in this order, until such time as a better one can be established by the rediscovery of the book itself, and with a common title for everything, *Anatomy*. This is only our intuition, our suggestion, although there is sound reasoning behind it. Anyone who agrees with it, can follow it; but if not, he can continue to read his books in their individual and corrupt state and use them in the traditional way. The value of our suggestion will not escape anyone, should they wish to use it; but it will not put pressure on anyone, should they prefer to do without it.[152] I just wanted to warn the careful reader, and offer others food for thought, and encourage scholars to seek out Greek texts of Hippocrates and Galen, and edit and publish them. In this regard, I would pay a great tribute to the very learned Agostino Gadaldino, our onetime friend in Italy with the Giuntas, as well as to Niccolò Machello and Gianbattisa Rasario, had they sent to press the works of Galen in Greek that they translated.[153] I would like old manuscripts to be brought out of domestic shadows and darkened places into the middle of the action and the arena of vigorous scholarly debate, and into the full light of day. They would then be read to the greatest and fullest satisfaction of men who know Greek

Restoration of Hippocrates' and Galen's works.

and Latin./21r Gadaldino translated *The Anatomy of Muscles; The Anatomy*   Gadaldino.
of Nerves; The Anatomy of the Organs of Voice; and *Medical Statements in*
Plato's Timaeus; Machello the beginning of Galen's first commentary on the   Machello.
first book of Hippocrates' *Epidemics;* Rasario the seventh and eighth com-   Rasario.
mentary by Galen, and half of the sixth, on the sixth book of Hippocrates'
Epidemics, and the three commentaries by Galen on Hippocrates' book *On*
Humours; and with greater hope of more to come.[154]

After we had edited Hippocrates' *Anatomy*, we next wrote for Conrad   The book *Rare*
Gessner a book divided into four sections, *An Enquiry into Rare Animals and*   *Animals.*
Plants. In the first we spoke about quadrupeds, in the second about birds, in
the third about fishes, and the fourth about rare plants. We also wrote to him
about them later.[155] You will find everything, together with illustrations, in
his books on animals, except for the hartebeest, the Barbary sheep, the long-
tailed Arabian sheep, the pod of the grains of paradise [*aframomum melegu-*
eta], the Jerusalem palms and both kinds of ilex.[156] We sent him descriptions
and drawings of all these a little before his death, after he had published his
animal books.[157] William Seres, the London printer, has printed it /21v alongside this tract of ours.

We also wrote a book on British dogs for the same man, who was a very   Praise of Gesner.
dear friend while he lived and whose unexpected death on December 13,
1565, so afflicted my spirit that it was not assuaged by the passage of time
(which should be a healer of the bitterest grief even in weak women).[158]
Indeed, it increased more and more by thinking about it, not just because of
the marriage of our minds (which should constitute the strongest relationship) or his attitude to me but inspired just as much by his unblemished goodness and his remarkable knowledge and wide reading, for which I not only
liked but loved him a great deal.[159] But what can you do against fate, since life   Fate is
and death exist by the law of nature, and both dying and living are ours,   immutable.
indeed since in living we also die? What can you do against the common
accidents of mortality? Tears are no use, nor can the fates be moved; and
there is but one end of us all: we have lived. We should bear with moderation
what is unavoidable. It should be sufficient solace that he had a good life and
a good death, and enjoyed a good reputation everywhere for his singular gifts
of mind, with which he greatly benefitted his state; and would have done so
with greater glory, had fate permitted.[160] He rests in peace, a man of felicity,   The peace of
goodness and justice, away from the turbulence and miseries of this life   death.
which we /22r mortals left behind (who largely take the same view of right
and wrong as he did) still endure unhappily and in sadness, even if we are
raised to wealth and splendour; and despite the fact that he who has the greatest wealth may also enjoy the greatest authority. Indeed, should one consider   Human life's
more deeply the iniquitous condition of living, one might certainly under-   calamity.
stand, as Posidippus, the comic poet from Cassandreia, used to say, that it is
preferable never to have been born, or, once born, to perish as quickly as
possible.[161] How filled with evils it is, how much at the mercy of events, how

exposed to the slings and arrows of fortune, grief drives me to declare in a few words, although our daily round teaches us very fully. To begin at the very first moments of our life, even if you yourself are unaware, who does not observe that Nature wanted the new-born to have crying and wailing, and that the sense of happiness, which is detected in laughter, was not introduced before the fortieth day? We are all brought into the light with these beginnings, and the passage of what follows is common to all. Should you wish to look back at the enormity of misfortunes and sadnesses that loom over you, this provides certainly constant and substantial material for misery, a great reason for tears. Such is the fear that things might change, or Fortune ruin everything, that it is perpetually with us. Fires consume this man, murder removes that one; the waves engulf another, yet another falls victim to a falling roof-tile; one man is finished off by a storm, another swallowed up by the gaping earth; a third dies from a snake-bite, yet another in a headlong fall. /22v Laborious poverty drives one man to his daily task; restless ambition plagues another; another is afraid for the luxurious riches (which are simply the playthings of Fortune) that he had prayed for, and struggles because his prayers have been answered, as Seneca writes.[162] This man is oppressed by anxiety, another by the hostility of others; a third is tormented by the effort required to maintain his wealth; another feels harassed by the many who crowd round his door or accost him in the street. This man is oppressed by winter's cold, this man by summer's heat. Thirst is what troubles one man, hunger another; this man is driven mad by foolish love, his neighbour wastes away through biting envy. This man grieves at his possession of a wife and family, this one, contrariwise, at his loss, which shows extremely well the vanity of life. An unfulfilled hope in deceitful Fortune disturbs this man, this man is bowed down under the weight of a Fortune whose munificence he had never expected. She raises one man up, and puts down another; this man starts a fight and another goes to law for things that are of only passing importance or will never amount to anything more than pinchbeck as if [the contest were] for hearth and home.[163] So, as Diogenes the sage used to say, to reach a proper attitude to life sometimes requires to be dragged along, at others to be convinced by reason.[164] In short, to stop trying to measure this piece of string, there is nothing in life that is not tainted with gall.[165] So, if reason cannot put a stop to the miseries of human life, neither will Fortune, and life itself will end before the occasion for grieving does; so great are the cares of mankind, so empty the world. Indeed, when you have been for a long while tossed about by the storms of this life, enduring many dangers, just when you are hoping to spend very pleasantly what remains of your life, /23r illnesses (of which Pliny writes that there are more than three hundred) ambush our lives and a sad old age creeps upon you.[166] Finally you will be forced to meet your death as the bonds of nature give way; a truly marvellous reward for having lived. Yet this is a fixed rule of Nature and never fails. Indeed, things

Misfortune.

Reasons should rule in life, otherwise death.

Diseases.

Old age.
Life's short span.

are so ordered that Nature gives us a hotel to visit, not a house to live in. Because the elements of our constitution are easily corruptible, and their bonds easily dissolved by the slightest accident, Nature has circumscribed for us a brief course of life, so that no one can know or discover whether his body will last even until nightfall, let alone for a year. Yet, although it is short (for all human life is but a dot in time, as Plutarch says in *Bringing up Children*), I would be ready to embrace it with greater equanimity if it were pleasant, happy or, at any rate, free from troubles.[167] But since living is merely the prolongation of a period of great unhappiness, weighed down with human calamity, and Fortune's plaything, why should we make so much of it? Old Cato was wise in my opinion when he wrote: 'Were God to grant me the opportunity to throw aside my years and become a child again, mewling in its cot, I would vigorously refuse, and I would not wish to be recalled from the finishing line to the starting gate when my race has been run.[168] For what is the advantage of living? Is it not, rather, hard labour? Certainly, any benefit, should there be one, would be either too great or too small. I take no pleasure in bewailing our life, as many philosophers have done. I am not ashamed to have lived in such a way /23v that I do not think I have been born in vain. And I depart this life, as if from a hospice, not a home. For Nature has given us a hotel to visit, not a house to live in. Oh for that glorious day, when I go to join that great council and company of souls, and depart from this crowded sordidity!' Thus Cato the Elder. Therefore, in the perpetual fragility of our body, in the brief and bitter span of our life, amid the turbulent storms of Fortune, I persuade myself that our dearest friend, Conrad Gessner, was fortunate to leave the land of the living as he did. Assuredly, Death took counsel on his behalf and did not bear a grudge against him but loved him when it snatched him away from so many evils; indeed, it would have hated him, had it kept him alive. Death's charity is visible in the fact it did not remove him, like Socrates and Phocion, by hemlock, or like Lucius Seneca through a prince's wrath, or like Epaminondas through a capital trial, or like Scipio through exile, Aristides through the envy of the people and Themistocles through poison, or like Diogenes by a squid, Aeschylus by a tortoise, Sophocles by a grape pip, Euripides by being torn to pieces by dogs, and Homer ravaged by hunger.[169] Instead, he died a natural death, amid universal gratitude, and after only the briefest of illnesses.[170] And, since we must die sometime, what does it matter to us whether we meet our fate sooner or later? No-one should refuse to endure a fate that we all must suffer. We should seek /24r only to have a good death. And a good death is the end of a good life. We should not be broken by a desire for a life that, when it is with us, afflicts us with pains, and when it leaves, frees us from an entirety of troubles, which are so numerous in life that they assuredly cannot be numbered. Yet no one dies willingly, and I do not know why we are so complacent, since we miserable souls are an exemplar of weakness, the prey of time, the plaything of Fortune, the image

Life's inconveniences.

Eternity desirable.

Fortunate death of Gesner.

of inconstancy, weighed down with envy and calamity, and all that is left is phlegm and bile, or something even nastier. Thus, even if we ourselves have no truck with Fortune's blandishments, we may decide that Fortune dealt kindly with Gessner since he can rightly be called not unhappy. Indeed, he should be universally termed most fortunate for that very reason and especially because he strove against Fortune and against the brevity of our mortal life though his goodness, his writings and his achievements (which are the work of virtue). In this way, he extended his reputation by his deeds, and his mind remains immortal and immutable, though once housed in a mortal and feeble body. He left behind for posterity the memory of a virtuous life, so that he can live on after his death, and still remain among mankind after his decease; for though the path of life may be short, the path of glory is everlasting.[171] Just as it is a great thing to lead a blameless life, it is the greatest of all to surround oneself for all eternity with the glory of outstanding talents and superlative achievements. The former can never be snatched away in life, the latter not even in death. /24v So there is, after all, no more cause for weeping if human afflictions do not carry us off, but rather cause for rejoicing.[172] He laid aside his life, he did not lose it; he set down his spirit, and gained glory, which can always be greater after death than in life, when envy departs and immediate personal impressions fall away. But I am a man, and I know that nothing human is alien to me.[173] I feel the tight bonds of affection, and because of his sweetness of character, now lost to fate, I cannot release them at will. But I shall summon my mind back from mourning to the books from which I departed, in order to see whether a change of theme produces a different state of mind, so that study and turning my thoughts away from sadness can create a distraction, something that time alone cannot do.

British Dogs.   I now return to the book on dogs where my digression began. In it we explained the breeds, use and nature, the differences and habits of British dogs (in which I included Scottish). When Conrad Gessner wrote asking me to do this, we wrote to him first in a rather crude and hurried manner, with a rough and unpolished outline. Since he was more delighted with this than I had imagined, he promised to publish it swiftly in the abridgement of *On Animals* that he entitled *Illustrations*, where he deals with Scottish dogs in the second section on domesticated animals.[174] Since this still was not entirely satisfactory to me, I wrote back asking him not to arrange for the book to go to press; I would produce a better revision for him. This is why we wrote /25r our book to please him, and gave it the title of *British Dogs, for Gessner*, published by William Seres in 1570, since fate would not allow it to be published by such a great scholar.[175]

The Agreement of British Words.   After that had been finished, we wrote another little book about British words, in which we showed how our British tongue agrees with Greek and Latin; for many of our race derive their origin from the Greeks, since Brutus the Trojan, and before him Albania, daughter of the king of Greece, are recorded to have lived after the original fathers of our race, and later the Romans muddled everything with their own pronunciation.[176]

We also wrote *A Londoner, or Two Books on the Antiquity of the University of Cambridge*, which, after being earlier attacked by a certain Oxonian, we perforce had printed at London in May, 1568, by Henry Bynneman.[177] We showed there that Cambridge University is far older than Oxford, and Oxford far younger than the Oxonian wanted; and that it was a fraudulent fiction to take that university back to Alfred as its founder, and still more to the men of Cricklade.[178] In refuting the diatribe of the Oxonian in which he held a different view, we also showed additionally in our books how a comparison with our own allowed everyone to see how far he had missed his aim. We have enlarged them, and submitted them anew to the press, along with a third edition of our *Method of Healing*.[179] There is no further point in concealing our authorship, /25v since the whole affair is known to everybody, although we carefully pretended it was not.

We also composed two books on the history of Cambridge University from the foundation of the city. In Book I we described how the city once was, its founders and the ruinous episodes of strife that it suffered. In Book II we showed how the city is today and has been in our lifetime.[180] We wrote this and *A Londoner* while we were building our College in Cambridge.

We wrote also a book on British baths. In it we explained the nature, use and effects of baths, and their discovery; with a preface on the kindness of Nature to this island, not just in the fertility of the soil and in the general universal affluence, but also in what conduces most to human health.[181]

There was also a single book on ancient towns, where we explain what they once were, what those that have not yet disappeared were called both now and in the past, with a mention too of those that have ceased to be.[182]

A single book in Greek on *Works of Galen no longer extant*, together with arguments drawn from Galen so that, even if we do not have the actual books, we have their arguments, as with those of Trogus in Justin.[183] We have not yet published them, but we will do so soon.

Finally, this single book on our own books, whose general argument and reason for writing you have at the beginning of this book. William Seres /26r the printer published this in 1570.

We also created for our own use an apparatus and almost a commentary for a future edition of all the works of Galen in Greek (for they are extremely corrupt), if the fates allow, partly from old books we have in Britain, partly from old books in Italy where I travelled almost everywhere in 1543 to see national characteristics, cities and libraries.[184] These [readings] came principally from books in the Library of Ss. Giovanni e Paolo at Venice, which were good but obviously badly preserved and maltreated. Many had been badly rubbed in many places, especially in *The Use of Parts*, so that not even

Londoner.

Cambridge History.

British Baths.

Ancient Towns.

Galen's Books no longer extant.

An Autobibliography.

Editing Galen's works.

Italian Libraries.

traces of the true reading still remained.[185] [Figure 9] Others were taken from books in the Libraries of S. Mark's and of S. Antonio in the same city, and in that of S. Giovanni in Verdara at Padua, which were given, if my memory does not deceive me, by Bessarion, a Greek and Patriarch of Constantinople.[186] Ditto from books in the public library of the Medici at S. Lorenzo in Florence, where, among many Greek texts, we left behind Dioscorides' *Medical Experience with Simple and Compound Drugs*, also a single book of Galen on *Urines*; Galen's commentaries on Hippocrates, *Epidemics* III; the single book of *My own Books*; the single book of *The Order of my own Books*.[187] There was also a work in two books on *The Composition of Drugs, by Site* (as it is called today),/26v which was bought by Angelo Poliziano (the teacher of Pope Leo) while at his little estate at Fiesole on April 25th, 1497, as anyone can discover who wants to transcribe and edit them or seeks to emend the writings of Galen from them.[188] He can do this thanks to the generosity of that most noble prince Cosmo de' Medici, always most keen to help students of literature, whom I mention so often since I myself can never do so enough.[189] Indeed, whatever words I use to praise cannot fail to be outdone by his virtuous actions; such is the benevolence of the Duke and his family towards literature and scholarship, and his kindness to his guests. Fiesole is an ancient Italian town, whose mayor Sallust calls '*Faesulanus*'.[190] They say that Florence grew out of its ruins, like the new city from the devastated remains of old Rome.[191] It is a mile and a half, or roughly two thousand paces, from Florence to the North (if I remember correctly), on the top of a mountain.[192] Because of its reputation in antiquity we visited it in 1543, when there was a festival and fair. Of the books in the library of the Duke of Urbino we have chosen to mention a few. It was built and assembled by Federico, Duke of Urbino, where, among other rarities, there is a copy of Galen's *Drugs easy to Hand*.[193] Among those in the Vatican Library, which is filled more with Greek than Latin, we saw manuscripts of Augustine, *On /27r the Trinity*, Thomas Aquinas, and Publius Ovid's *Metamorphoses* in Greek. There was also Galen, *On Bandages*; and a Greek collection of words old and new.[194] I mention these in particular because there were few books in our day at Ferrara, in the library of S. Domenico, which Celio Calcagnini had supplied with many volumes, or at SS. Angeli, which Ercole, first Duke of Ferrara had built;[195] in Florence at S. Marco and S. Maria, and at Bologna at S. Domenico and S. Salvatore.[196] There were absolutely none at the library at Siena which Pope Pius III had built at the cathedral.[197] Siena, a now famous Tuscan town in Italy, was, I declare. built in 362 BC by Brennus the Englishman, the chief of the Gauls (to whom many towns in Italy they say owe their existence) and was named (I think) after the island of Sena in our Britain.[198] Nor was there anything memorable in the libraries just mentioned except for a manuscript of Pliny in philosophy at S. Maria in Florence; and. in theology, one of Esdras, written, they say, by the prophet himself, at S. Domenico in Bologna.[199] When I say books, I largely mean Greek manuscripts, for they were my main interest. In the

---

Marginal notes (left column):

The Laurentian Library.

Politian.

Cosmo de' Medici's kindness.

Fiesole.

The library at Urbino.

Thomas Aquinas, Ovid.

The Ferrara library.

The Siena library, Siena.

The library at S. Maria. Esdras. The library at Bologna. The restoration of Pisa university.

university of Pisa, long deserted but restored in 1543 by the good offices of
Duke Cosmo de' Medici /27v and provided with new lecture halls, there was
no library as far as I know; but there could well be if it pleases their extremely
learned prince, if it has not already happened between then and now.[200] Outside libraries, I examined books at Pisa with Corti and Pontremoli, and at
Ferrara with Antonio Musa Brasavola, Niccolò Bonacciuoli, Ippolito Canano
and Giambattista Canano.[201] I went to see these men for medicine, just as I
consulted Guarino, the most Latinate of men, and Antimaco, the Greek professor of humanity at the latter university, for the new theory about the pronunciation of Greek and Latin.[202] I observed them diligently using the old   The pronunciation
pronunciation (like other Greeks from Greece itself in lectures and in divine   of Greek and
offices at Venice).[203] Likewise at Padua, Lazzaro Bonamico, at Bologna   Latin.
Achille Bocchi and Pompilio Amuseo and in Venice the celebrated Giambattista Egnazio.[204] At Rome, because it was the vacations or holidays at the   Rome.
old and new Sapienza when I was there, I heard no one lecturing.[205] I just
saw the ruins of ancient Rome and whatever other memorable monuments
worth looking at had survived, which were many; and I visited the Vatican
library (which contained Greek and Hebrew manuscripts in two rooms, and
Latin in a third). We have already spoken about its manuscripts. In Germany,
too, Melanchthon, Joachim Camerarius, Sebastian Münster /28r (with all of
whom we were on friendly terms) and all those at Louvain whom I knew and
heard (including Jeremias Drivère van Brachel) used the old pronunciation.[206] What pronunciation Erasmus used Cantabrigians knew well (for he
spent many years among them), and Levinus and Hieronymus Froben (with
whom he lodged) also told me.[207] But on that we have written substantially   *The pronunciation
in another book entitled *The new Pronunciation and Writing of Greek and*   *of Greek and*
Latin.[208] In it we argue that one should not use the new modern pronuncia-   *Latin.*
tion that has been proposed, and even less the spelling, taking into account
the great antiquity, novelty, difficulty, hardness, boorish rusticity, inconsis-
tency, absurdity, juvenile error, unsuitability, laughability, despicable nature,
rustic simplicity, childish puerility, fraud, trickery, the habits of the wise,
peaceful tranquillity amid its turbulent doctrines, the pleasant smoothness of
the old pronunciation, the temporal spread of the topic, the age of those who
use this awful sound, frivolity, the authority of approved authors, the weight
or lack of it of individuals, the emptiness of the argument, received custom,
diversity, common usage, popular feeling, insolence, vainglory, emulation
and contentiousness of teachers, fickleness, offensiveness, Scotism and
logic chopping, mutual borrowing, the abandonment of understanding,
usage and authority of teachers, and even moral turpitude.[209] I did this can-
didly and in the fullness of charity, not without respect for my betters, and
with benevolence /28v towards those who use it, as well as offering sound
advice, but leaving it to everyone to follow whatever conclusion they wished.
When we first projected this autobibliography, we resolved to follow this
[question] up during our travels through Italy, Upper and Lower Germany
and France, where they used the old pronunciation. But when it entered my

mind to list our books here, not just describe those that were complete, we brought it out of its [hiding] place and put it on the side [of our desk]; we also returned to the apparatus of readings (the start of our digression) for a future edition of all the extant works of Galen.[210] It is most often in my prayers that I should see it finished and complete before my own end (I am now in my sixtieth year and senior but not senile), either through my own efforts or those of another. [Galen's writings] are in a dreadful state, but more through misfortune than through their own failings. For they display genius. That is why I would wish, all the more, for everyone with an interest in medicine and who owns ancient Greek copies to work together to bring this task to a conclusion for the common use of all, and for all owners to bring their own copies into the light. For it has always seemed to be a better and more assured method of study to unearth from the authorities in any branch of learning whatever should be learned, and to search for it, no matter what language it is written in, both because water is best drunk from the actual spring, and because through regular use it makes the author a friend. Just as /29r everyone is more fluent, more self-assured and always self-consistent in his own tongue, which is obvious, so every language has its own idiom and secrets, which, when translated into another language, do not always keep the same emphasis or an equal charm. (Not to mention that translators sometimes fail to grasp the meaning, sometimes nod, do not keep the meaning of the text, tone down a purple passage, make a slip (for we are all human), and are so keen on variety that the result is not only obscurity, but also ambiguity.)[211] That is why from the beginning of our studies we made up our mind to read what was originally written in Latin in Latin, and Greek in Greek, so that in making our judgments, we might trust ourselves rather than others, and manage everything with a more reliable methodology and a better sense of the essentials. Everyone flies to a Latin edition, no-one takes up a Greek, either because there is a greater profit [for publishers] in Latin because of the large number of Latinate students, or because everyone grudges showing the world what he has, or because their own Greek copies are destroyed in the process of translation to prevent their errors from being detected, and, perhaps, their own texts from being translated by others. For everyone today is keen to take his sickle to another's harvest as he sees fit, something of which I do not approve.[212] I would think them better scholars and likely to win greater universal thanks if they were to publish the texts they own in both Greek and Latin, as many scholars do.[213] The result would be that medical schools would flourish with consummate learning, the health of mortals would be conserved,/29v and life, which is otherwise short and unhealthy, would be preserved for a long while with its strength intact, which should be the prayer of all doctors. My dear Hatcher, you now have your wish. You have the little tract on my own books which you have extorted from me by your smooth eloquence before it was really ready. Should you find it pleasing, that is a bonus; but if not, at least I wanted to fall in with your wishes as a friend. We have produced it without the need for lengthy prefaces or flashy titles,

An exhortation to edit Galen's works.

Books should be read in the original language.

first because I dislike them, and would not want you to think that I would bring just anything to your attention, and secondly because the olden days did not use this sort of writing. Galen simply entitles his books *For Piso, For Pamphilianus, For Glauco, For Thrasybulus, For Eugenianus, For Theo, For Bassus*; and Cicero *For Atticus, For Herennius, For my Son Marcus*; and

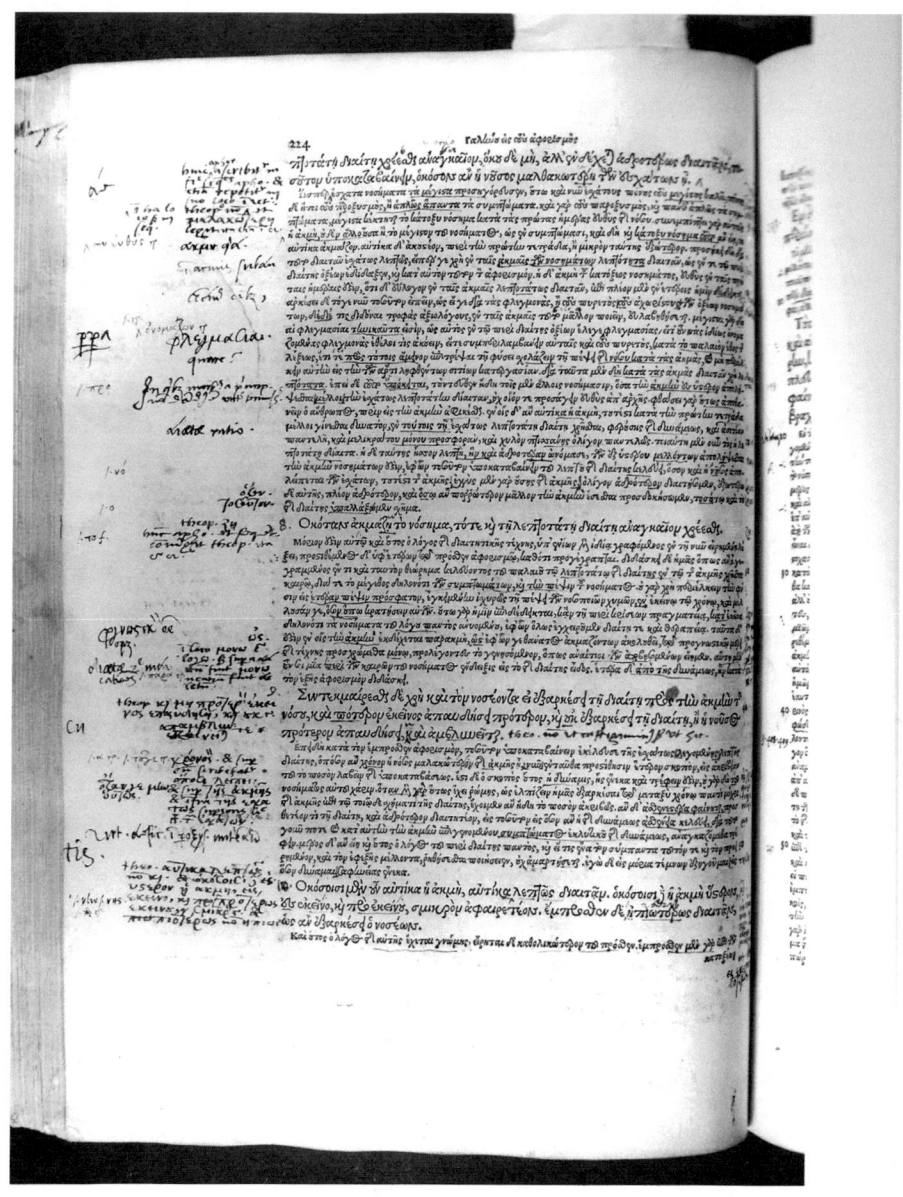

Figure 9   Caius' annotated copy of Galen, Eton College Library, Fc 2,6–8, Tome V, p. 224.The varied handwriting and the colour of the ink indicate notes written by Caius over a long period, including transcriptions from MSS and his own corrections.

several others among the ancients do likewise.[214] Such an argument, I know, cannot fail to meet with your approval as a lover of Antiquity.

End of the autobibliography of John Caius, Briton./30r

This last part of our book dealt with unpretentious titles; now, dear Hatcher, take this as a sort of epilogue, an organized list of books we either edited or composed.

The Method of Healing, two books.*
The British Ephemeral Fever, two.*
The British Ephemeral Fever, for the People of Britain, one book.*
The Antiquity of Cambridge University, two.*
The History of Cambridge University, two.*
British Dogs, one.*
Rare Animals and Plants, one.*
The Agreement of the British Vocabulary [with Greek and Latin], one.
British Baths, one.
The Ancient Towns of Britain, one.
My Autobibliography, one.*
The New Pronunciation and Spelling of Greek and Latin, one.*
The Annals of the London College of Physic, one.*
The Annals of Gonville and Caius College, one.*
A Summary of Erasmus' True Theology, one.

Commentaries or notes

On Cornelius Celsus' *Eight Books of Medicine*.[215] /30v
On Scribonius Largus' book on the *Composition of Drugs*.
On the Complete Works of Framingham.
On the Nine Books of Galen's *Anatomical Procedures*.* [CULAdv]
On the two books of his *Movement of Muscles*.* [CULAdv]
On the six books of *The Preservation of Health*.*
On the single book of *Barley Gruel*.*
On the single book of *The Small Ball*.
On the single book of *For Thrasybulus*.
On the single book of *Bones for Beginners*.*

Our translations

The Opinions of Hippocrates and Plato, Book 1.*
Galen's My own Books, one book.*
The Order of my own Books, one book.*
Diet in Acute Diseases, one.*
Nicephorus Callistus, *Confession in Prayer*, one.

Chrysostom, *Manner of Prayer*, one.
Erasmus' *Paraphrase of the Epistle of St. Jude*, one.

Books involving textual correction[216]

Galen's *Anatomical Procedures*, nine books.*
The Movement of Muscles, two.*
Bones for Beginners, one.*
The Composition of Drugs, seventeen books /31r
The Properties of Simples, eleven
The Opinions of Hippocrates and Plato, nine.*
The Method of Healing, fourteen
My own Books, one.*
The Order of my own Books, one.*
The Preservation of Health, six.*
The Small Ball, one.
For Thrasybulus, one.
Barley Gruel, one.*
The Rationale for Diet in Acute Diseases, one.*
Substitute Drugs, one.*
The Seven-month Child, one.*
Humours, one.
A Short Description of the Doctrines of Hippocrates, one.*
The Use of Parts, seventeen.[217]
Affected Parts, complete with summaries of each book.
The Difference between Fevers, one.
The Difference between Diseases, one.
The Causes of Diseases, one.
The Causes of Symptoms, three.
The Temporal Stages of Illness, one
The Property of Purgative Drugs, one.
Who, How and When to be Purged, one.
Hippocrates' *Anatomy*, one. /31v
Galen's *Dissection of Muscles*, one.
Galen's *Dissection of Nerves*, one.
The eight books of Celsus' *Medicine*.
The single book of Scribonius' *The Composition of Drugs*.

Books we discovered

The Opinions of Hippocrates and Galen, Book I.*
Coma, a single book in Greek.*
Hippocrates*, On Drugs*, in Greek, one

Part of Galen's *The Use of Parts*, Book VII, in Greek.*
The missing bit of *Barley Gruel*.[218]

We have decided to write a history of Norwich, as well as to edit the complete works of Galen, unless the fates intervene and break the thread of our life.

This list, which was [originally] left out, should be added to the last line of the text so that the book ends there.

End of the list of books with which John Caius, Briton, involved himself. /32v

Index of the contents of this small book

The number marks the folio, the letter the page

B

Notes

1 The edition of 1570 bears the Latin title *De libris suis, His Books*, but Caius himself in the opening title inside and in the colophon used the more elegant *De libris propriis, My/his own Books*. Whether Caius changed his mind when passing his manuscript to the publisher or Seres misremembered when designing the title page is not clear; the latter is more likely in view of the fact that *De libris propriis* was the Latin version given by Fichard and, with a change in word order, by Caius himself to the title of the Greek tract by Galen that served as a model.

2 Thomas Hatcher, d. 1583, son of John Hatcher, later regius professor of Physic at Cambridge, was himself a Cambridge don, a friend of Archbishop Parker and of others known to Caius, to whose College library he donated a Greek MS of the Gospels, MS 403/412 and probably the Latin bestiary MS 372/621. He also composed a poem for the ceremony of laying the foundation stone of the College (Venn (1904: 14): Beer (2004)). Thomas' brother, Michael Hatcher, acquired in 1540 a copy of some Galenic treatises that had once belonged to Vesalius in Padua (now London, Wellcome Library, EPB 1536), probably from an Englishman who had been in Padua or perhaps directly on a brief (and unrecorded) visit there.

3 For Gessner, see above, pp. 15–18. He may have made the request to allow him to include an up-to-date list of Caius' writings in one of the editions of his *Biblioteca Universalis*, first published in 1545, and revised and subsequently enlarged. Caius' name does not appear in the first edition of the *Bibliotheca universalis* (Gessner 1545), but a list of his writings appears in the *Epitome* of 1555 (Lycosthenes and Simler 1555: sig. q2v) and in the Appendix to the enlarged edition of the *Bibliotheca* of the same year (Gessner 1555: 92v).

4 This rhetorical opening has many parallels in Galen, who often insisted that his books had, so to speak, been extorted from him by friends and colleagues.

5 See above, note 3.

6 Hatcher had edited the poems and other writings of Walter Haddon in 1567, and was to publish a revised and enlarged collection in 1576. Hatcher (1567) contains a liminary poem by John Friar, M.D., identified by Lees (1967: 84) with the Paduan contemporary of Caius, d. 1563, but more likely to have been his namesake, also a Paduan-trained physician, who practised at Godmanchester and was a Fellow of the London College of Physicians. See Woolfson (1998: 238); White (2004).

7 I.e. in 1531/2, but in the earlier account (1552: 3 = 5 R.), Caius says that he was 'of the age of twenty yeres'.

8 Ibid., 6 = 5 R., Caius names the friend as John Groome, a Cambridge B. A., 'a young man in yeres, but in witte & learnyng for his tyme, of great expectation.' He is probably the John Groome who took his B.A. in 1529–30 rather than the scholar of the same name who graduated in 1536–37 and became briefly a Fellow of St John's. The elder Groome owned the two-volume Aristotle (Basle: J. Bebel 1531), which Caius later owned and annotated in his Italian hand, particularly the zoological tracts in vol. I and the *Problems* in vol. II, now Gonville and Caius College Library, G.32.4–5. Nicephorus Callistus, fl. 1320, was a Byzantine cleric and historian, remembered today largely for his *Ecclesiastical History*, but the author also of religious works (Jugie 1931, but with no mention of this tract). Both Callistus and Caius are arguing against the doctrine that only the oral confession of sins to a priest is valid.

9 Caius was already developing his links with the court and capital, although he does not name the friend. Erasmus had published in 1525 an edition and the first Latin translation of the two homilies on prayer ascribed to the Byzantine patriarch, St John Chrysostom (347–407) (*Patrologia graeca* 50: 775–86). Caius may have used this edition, Basle: Froben, 1525, or a later printing. For the importance of prayer in Erasmus' theology, see Pabel (1997).

10 For the recipient, Alderman Augustine Stiward of Norwich, see above, p. 41, note 6. Erasmus' *Ratio verae theologiae*, 'the true and redye way to reade the scripture', was first published at Louvain in 1518 by T. Martens, but Caius may well have used the enlarged edition, Basle: Froben, 1520 (English translation by Grant 1998).

11 This is a sideswipe at the Lutheran ideas that had flourished in Cambridge in the 1530s, and were later to inform the evangelical puritanism that Caius so disliked. For his theological views in the context of Cambridge, see Appendix II.

12 Erasmus' *Paraphrase on the Epistle of Jude* was first published by Martens at Louvain in 1520 but became more accessible in the several editions put out from 1521 by Froben in Basle (English translation by Bateman 1993). None of the copies of the 1521 and 1522 editions of the *Paraphrases in omnes epistulas* in Gonville and Caius College Library was owned by Caius.

13 Venn and Venn (1922: 2, 171).

14 Shown by the list of his library (Smith 1974: 29–31, with the commentary, below, notes 15–20).

15 These poems illustrate Framingham's mastery of all the classical Latin metres: *On Consolation* in elegiac couplets, *Laurence* and *Ecpyrosis* in hexameters, *Idolatry* in a complex metre used particularly in Antiquity for satire, and *Epigrams* in a variety of metres. His writings are typical of the period in melding ancient and modern, and in using classical Latin genres and examples to illustrate Christian concerns of the day.

16 St Laurence was martyred in 258, traditionally by being roasted on a gridiron. Caius quotes the opening lines, which suggest the following scenario: Laurence, devoted to a life of poverty among the poor, is betrayed by the crafty Detius (or the craftsman Detius, cf. *Acts* 19, 24), and handed over to a raging mob. He achieves glory by his martyrdom, whereas his tormentor or prosecutor, Mezentius, ends in Hell. The names of Detius and Mezentius are not given in earlier accounts of the martyrdom. Detius recalls (and may be a copyist's or printer's error for) the persecuting emperor Decius (d. 251), who in some late martyrologies, including the widely read *Legenda aurea* of Jacopo de Voragine (d.1298), is named as the judge who condemned Laurence to death (Sollerius et al. 1867: 140–1, 410, 518–19). The name Mezentius was also borne by the bloodthirsty and impious Etruscan ruler slain by Aeneas at the end of Vergil's *Aeneid*, Book 10.

17 The burning of Sodom, whose 'men were wicked, great sinners against the Lord', is described briefly in *Genesis* 19, 24–28.

18 The glyconic metre, a complex mixture of short and long syllables, ⌣- l – ⌣- l⌣- or – l – ⌣-l⌣-, was taken over from Greek into Latin by poets such as Catullus and Horace, e.g. Horace, *Odes* 1, 5, 8 and 16: *emirabitur insolens;* and: *vestimenta maris deo.* A choriambus is a mixture of two long and two short syllables: – ⌣-.

19 Earlier (1552: 5 = 6 R.) he mentioned that Framingham had originally composed two books of epigrams, of which only one remained, and was dedicated to Caius himself.

20 Caius' comments both assist others to understand these highly sophisticated poems and serve his own purposes as a test of his own skills. The alternative possibility, that Caius is delighted to put his learning on display for others to review, makes a less attractive contrast between the two.

21 More details of this misfortune are given in *The Sweat* (Caius 1552: 6 = 7–8 R.). For the Cambridge links of those involved, see above, p. 7.

22 For his links with Parker, see above, p. 7; Grafton (2017); for Guest (1514–77), formerly Parker's domestic chaplain), see Freeman (2004).

23 A good example of Caius' fallible erudition. Tacitus, *Agricola* 18, mentions the annihilation of a Roman detachment by what in modern editions is rightly given as *Ordovicum civitas*, 'the community of the Ordovices', a tribe in North Wales. However, Polydore Vergil in his *Historia anglica* II, 6, misunderstood '*civitas*' as 'town', and by adding a preliminary 'N', identified it with Norwich and transferred the tribe to Norfolk. Venta Icenorum, recorded in the so-called Antonine Itinerary, *Iter Britanniarum* 5 and 9, is identified with the Roman site at Caistor St Edmund, approximately three km from Norwich. The Latin name of Norwich is a later formation from the Anglo-Saxon 'Northwick', referring to the most northern of the three settlements on the river Wensum. Anglo-Saxon remains at Caistor suggest that the two sites existed independently.

24 In 1552 (1552: 7 = 8 R) Caius had described it as a book, 'the matere whereof rude and undigested lyeth by me, which at laisure I intende to polishe, and to make an end of that I have begunne.' The book was never finished or published.

25 Another work by Caius, referred to in the concluding list, above, p. 82, but now lost. Cf. his comments on early British towns in his *Antiquity* (1574: 48–50 = 40–41 R.). His unusual interest in urban history and topography, which predates that of John Stowe and other London historians, is clear in Book II of his *History of Cambridge University* (1574c: 115–21 = 93–97 R.); Nutton (2017b).

26 Caius (1544a), reprinted in R.

27 Smith (1979) remains fundamental for Galen's borrowings; for Celsus (fl. 30), see Mudry (1982: 63–8); Manetti and Roselli (1994a: 112–21); Serbat (1995: xxix–xxxi, liii–lvii). The surviving books of Oribasius (320–400) are largely extracts and abridgements of Galen; the *Sixteen Books* of Paul of Aegina (d. after 642) summarize much of Galen; Macrobius, fl. 400, devoted chs. 2–16 of Book V of his *Saturnalia* to a discussion of Vergil's debts to Homer. Caius owned copies of both Paul and Macrobius (Grierson 1978: 515, 516, nos. 31 and 55).

28 Comparison with Crato's version and with Da Monte's original (1558) bears out Caius' claim for a substantial reworking of an author whose lectures, when published later, show enormous learning but an inability to leave almost anything out.

29 Caius is referring to the publication of Da Monte's *Methodus medicinae universalis* in the two-volume edition of his *Opuscula*, edited by Girolamo Donzellini, Basle: P. Perna, 1558, rather than the separate earlier publication, Vienna: M. Zimmermann, 1553.

30 Cicero, *The Nature of the Gods* I, 120. Cicero (106–43 BC) prided himself on introducing Greek philosophy into Latin.

31 Respectively Galen V.181–805 K. (modern edition with English translation by P. De Lacy 1978–84); a lost work from his student period in Smyrna (fragments in Marra (1966)); and a second work from this Smyrna period, largely lost in Greek (Schrenk 1989) but surviving today in Arabic, see Walzer (1944); Walzer and Frede (1985: 49–106). Caius took his information about these lost works from Galen's *My own Books* 2, 2 and 5: XIX.16–17 K. = Boudon-Millot (2007: 140–1).

32 Galen, *My own Books* 2, 3: XIX, 16 K. = Boudon-Millot (2007: 140). Both were doctors active in the 140s and 150s. 'Empiricist' in this context means a follower of the so-called Empiricist school, Greek doctors who rejected any investigation into causation in favour of detailed recording of cases and the application of remedies judged successful in similar cases.

33 Cicero, *The Nature of the Gods* I, 120. Democritus (fifth century BC) and Epicurus (341–270 BC) were Greek philosophers who believed in a universe built up from atoms.

34 Cicero, *Timaeus* (fragmentary); *Duties* II, 16, 86 and 88 (although the extent of his borrowing from Panaetius, a Stoic philosopher (185–109 BC) is disputed); Cicero's debt to the philosophical writings of Xenophon (430–360? BC) is small (Powell 1995: 280–3). Caius will doubtless have been thinking of Cicero, *Cato the Elder, On Old Age* 22, 79–81, a long passage avowedly translated from Xenophon's *The Education of Cyrus*. Cicero's version of Xenophon's *Running the Household* survives only in a few fragments.

35 Caius now uses Cicero's own words (above, note 30) about others to describe his activities. His claim, *Letters to Atticus* XII, 52, 3, that his writings were mere copies, long interpreted as his confession of dependence on Greek authors, is mock modesty and not necessarily relating to his philosophy (Powell 1995: 8–9).

36 Cicero, *Letters to Atticus* II, 1, 1. Isocrates (436–338 BC) was an Athenian orator and writer.

37 Theophilus Protospatharius (seventh century), *The Fabric of the Human Body*, appeared in the original Greek in 1555 (Paris: G. Morel), but was also known to Caius in an earlier Latin version by the Paduan teacher Giunio Paulo Grassi (Venice: O. Scotus, 1536), on whom see below, p. 89. Caius' commented on Theophilus' dependence on Galen in a note on the cover of the 1555 edition, Gonville and Caius College Library, K.34.42.

38 That the two Roman comic playwrights, Plautus (d. 184 BC) and Terence (d. 159 BC) had borrowed from the Greek comedians Menander (344/3–292/1 BC) and Apollodorus of Carystus (around 290 BC) was known from their prefaces and other ancient comments, but in Caius' day only tiny fragments of the originals were known in Greek (Fraenkel 2007; Brown 2013).

39 Caius derived his knowledge of this passage from the Greek historian Alexander Polyhistor (fl. 40 BC) directly or indirectly from Cyril of Alexandria's treatise *Against the Emperor Julian* 4, 133, where the author is named as Zaras, not Zoras. Modern editors of the text of the fragments of Alexander (Jacoby 1940: 118, 1943: 296–7) prefer the reading as given by a slightly earlier author, Clement, *Miscellanies* 1, 70, 1, who uses the variant form 'Zaratus'. The name may be a muddled form of Zoroaster.

40 Solinus (c. 250 AD), the Latin writer of a popular handbook of geography, *Wonders of the* World 2, 18, cites a Bocchus (unknown, although possibly the earlier historian Cornelius Bocchus) for the story that Homer in his *Iliad* had taken over some of the verse prophecies of the Delphic Sibyl in which she had predicted the

events of the Trojan War. That the Sibyl had made such predictions was widely believed in Antiquity, see Pausanias, *Guide to Greece* X, 12, 1, and the link with Homer was a natural consequence of learned speculation that was widely believed in the Renaissance.

41   Book XXI of the *History of Rome* by Livy (59 BC–AD 17?) deals with the second Punic War. The Greek historian Polybius (200–118? BC) is only one of the sources used by this Latin author (Luce 1977: 178–80).

42   Maximus Planudes (c. 1260–1305) made a very loose Greek translation of the Latin *Distichs* (moralizing couplets) ascribed to a Dionysius Cato (Ortoleva 1992). They were widely used in Erasmus' edition of Cato, *Catonis disticha* (Louvain: T. Martens 1514 and other editions). Caius owned a copy of Erasmus' *Apothegms*, a very popular collection of short sayings first printed in 1531 (Basle: Froben) (Grierson 1978: 516, no. 62). Plutarch (before 50–120) and Athenaeus (around 200 AD) were Greek miscellaneous writers.

43   Caius here turns the tables on Crato for his own book (Crato 1555). See above, p. 39.

44   The legendary Athenian King Theseus found his way out of the Labyrinth of the Minotaur by following a thread from a ball given him by Ariadne.

45   Caius has misremembered: according to Hesiod, *Theogony* 669–673, Zeus, king of the Greek gods, called for the assistance of the Hundred-handed Ones to help him in his great battle against the Titans.

46   Oribasius of Pergamum (c. 325–400) wrote a series of encyclopedias, or collections of extracts, the largest and most important of which is his *Medical Collections*. A Latin translation was produced by G. B. Rasario (Venice: Aldus 1554; Basle: M. Isingrin 1557), and a Greek text of the two books of anatomical material (XXIV and XXV) was separately published by G. Morel in Paris (G. Morel: 1556).

47   French and Lloyd (1978). A full list of borrowings from Galen is given in the indexes to Raeder's edition of Oribasius (Raeder: 1928–1929).

48   Neither edition was ever published: the first treatise (XVIIIB, 926–1026 K.; Garofalo and Debru 2005) was not printed in Greek until the nineteenth century, although Gadaldino's Latin version was available from 1550 (Galen 1550). The second, II, 831–49 K., is given a modern edition by Garofalo and Debru (2008).

49   Hieronymus (2005: 357). See above, p. 58. '*Romana littera*', presumably as distinct from an English Gothic script. While Caius refers to some passages of Galen in his text, he does not mention Da Monte. Nor does he here acknowledge the second printing at Louvain (1556), which contains only Caius' name on the title page.

50   Earlier discussions on medical method had concentrated on the logical processes involved (Wear 1981), whereas Da Monte, Caius and Crato followed Galen in applying the idea of method more widely to all aspects of clinical medicine.

51   Neither in the English original nor in the expanded Latin (1552, 1556) does Caius expressly state that his description is an example of good method, although his Galenic arrangement of topics in both books would have been noted by fellow scholars.

52   Leonhard Fuchs (1501–1566) published a short introductory compendium to medicine in 1531, *Compendiaria ac succincta admodum in artem medendi. . . . introductio*. Hagenau: J. Secerius. The second enlarged edition appeared in 1541 under a different title: *Methodus seu ratio compendiaria cognoscendi veram solidamque medicinam*, Lyons: S. Gryphius, and subsequently elsewhere. His preface (1541: a2r–8v) discusses the meaning of method, and declares that he is summarising Galen in order to provide a solid guide through disputes and complexities. For Fuchs, see Brinckhus and Pachnicke (2001, with plates, pp. 75, 78).

53 Caius (1544b): Hieronymus (2005: 100–1b). His later notes on *Anatomical Pro-cedures* are in Cambridge, CUL, Adv.d.3.1. For the edition of *The Movement of Muscles*, see Rosa (1999, 2009). For Bonamico, who owned a substantial col-lection of medical texts and was a friend of many doctors, see Avesani (1969); Nutton (1987a: 54, 68); Piovan (1988). The MS is probably to be identified with Paris, BNF gr. 1849, a fourteenth-century MS, which was in Italy, and almost certainly in Venice, since it was the source of Bessarion's copy, before it became part of the Ridolfi collection, below, note 58 (Garofalo 1986–2000: XI; Rosa 2009: XVI–XVII).

54 For Gadaldino, O'Malley (1964: 102–6); Nutton (1987a: 54, 69); Pastore (1998); Garofalo (2004); Boudon-Millot (2007: ccxxvi).

55 Caius (1544b: I, 136). The house where they stayed, in the S.W. quarter of the town between one of the bridges and the Prato della Valle cannot as yet be identi-fied. If Caius lodged with Vesalius immediately he arrived in Padua, his reminis-cence would date the beginning of the *Fabrica* to 1539–40; for further evidence on the date, see Nutton (2017a: 33–4). For Vesalius' role in the revision of the anatomical tracts in the 1540–41 edition of Galen, see O'Malley (1964: 101–8). Caius (1544b: 287) approves of Vesalius' use of illustrations.

56 Fortuna (2012).

57 Caius' description '*falsae*' could indicate that these were 'forgeries', but he is probably contrasting them with '*verae lectiones*', ('good readings'). Caius says more at 1544b: I, 320, declaring that 'these manuscripts were untrustworthy'; and, 286, that at least some readings were copied 'from an old codex'. Rather than fragmentary codices or collections of excerpts, these notes are likely to be conjectures made by others, but included in the margin of a printed book.

58 Nutton (1987a: 51); Berlier (2011). For Bessarion and his library, Labowsky (1979); Märtl et al. (2013) The MS is now Venice, Biblioteca Marciana 279, copied by Johannes Rhosos for Bessarion (Garofalo 1986–2000: XII–XIV, and, for a significant reading, XI, n. 12).

59 Caius (1544b); Hieronymus (2005: 100–1b). It was prepared in two parts, each with a separate list of contents the first with a dedication to Henry VIII, the sec-ond to Sir Anthony Denny (1501–1549), the Royal Chamberlain. The texts and translations are respectively: (1544b) I,[3]8–336; I, 25-[3]6; II, 55–76 with Ber-lier (2011; I, 1–18); and 337–54 with De Lacy (1978: 31, 776–80); I, 18–24 = VII, 643–65 K.; I, 18–24 with Mewaldt (1915: xv, 181–94); II, 77–78 with Monfort (2000). Caius (1544b: II: kk3–4) says he was helped by a '*studiosus*', possibly Cornarius according to Monfort (2000: 462), but this is unlikely. Caius does not mention here that the second volume contains his Greek edition of *The Movement of Muscles* (1544b: II, 5–44), above, pp. 82–3.

60 Grassi (d. 1574) published his Latin version in 1537, entitled *De purgatoriis medicamentis*, as an annexe to his translation of Theophilus, *De humani corporis fabrica*, Venice: O. Scotus, 1536: 111–14. For the subsequent argument over this section between Leonhard Fuchs and Janus Cornarius, see Monfort (2000: 306). Grassi encouraged Caius to edit *Anatomical Procedures* (Caius 1557: *3).

61 Caius will have used the famous Vatican Ms, Urbinas gr. 64, then in Urbino, see above, p. 67. He was correct in his division at this point, although he failed to recognise the fragmentary character of this 'Hippocratic' text. His supposi-tion, that it was added at some later date in order to form a 'complete' Hip-pocrates, is an intelligent guess: it is not found in the other large medieval MSS of Hippocrates that foreshadow something like our modern Hippocratic Corpus, although it may have been included in the lost part of Vatican, gr. 276 (Schoene 1924).

62 For Clement and Linacre, see above, p. 9. Readings from both MSS are given in CUL Adv.: Clement's MS was probably his annotated copy (Gundert 2006); Linacre's MS is now Leiden, Vulcanianus 57 (Nutton 1987a: 84–5). Caius has here a curious, lapse of memory, for the college, was founded in 1518. (Clark 1964: 89, 376) and he was nine times President. The relevant section of the *Annals* was printed in Roberts (1912), with separate pagination.

63 Details in Venn (1912: 27–36); see also anon. (1959: I, 73–81); Brooke (1985: 64–7); Nickson (2005). The date 1570 is given in the *Errata* for an original 1569.

64 Printed respectively in Venn (1904): 1–174; and Caius (1574c = 1–114 R.); the section on Caius College occupies pp. 64–66 = 51–53 R. Caius implies that it was completed by 1570; but he (or someone else) clearly continued to add details at least of new Heads of Houses until 1573 (1574c: 4 = 4 R.).

65 Neither was published. Caius' later notes on *Anatomical Procedures* can be read in CULAdv and on *The Use of Parts* in EtonAdv I, 367r–566v, on which see Nutton (1987a), Berlier (2011).

66 At the end of the century, in 1594, the University of Salamanca banned the use of any anatomical text bar *The Use of Parts*, as the latter contained all the anatomy a doctor needed to know in a manner appropriate for practical therapy. This reflected the opinions of Luiz Mercado (1520–1606), as Chief Physician of Spain, a vigorous Galenist who had little time for Vesalian anatomy (Skaarup 2015: 82–3, 97).

67 Caius (1544a: 100–14 = 50–6 R.)

68 Caius uses the word '*natura*' three times in a single sentence with three different meanings: the natural world; what constitutes the human body; and Nature as a creative force. Galen waxes lyrical on the miracle of creation in the final book of T*he Use of Parts:* IV, 346–66 K. For the trope of anatomy as leading to self-knowledge, see Schupbach (1982: 66–71).

69 They are still lost in Greek, but a good medieval Arabic translation of the missing books was published by Max Simon (1906); English translation by Duckworth et al. (1962).

70 Ambrosio Calepino, *Lexicon, adauctum et recognitum denuo*. Haguenau: H. Granius, 1526, the standard Latin dictionary of the day. Caius, naturally, had his own copy, presumably of this edition (Grierson 1978: 514, no. 11), which he also cites in his copy of Theophilus, Gonville and Caius College Library, K.34.42, fol. 2, and that of Gessner's *Icones*, Gonville and Caius College Library, L. 19, 4, . 57. He made the same comment earlier in his notes to his edition, CULAdv. 9, as well as at EtonAdv I,K.5v where he discusses the problems of editing this text from 'mutilated codices', and hopes for the recovery of the lost books, just as those of Aristotle had been rediscovered in the first century BC. For Antonio Visconti (d. after 1436), see Pellegrin (1955), but this volume is not recorded in his collection. Cf. also the report by Leonhard Fuchs of the complete text of Galen's lost *Demonstration* in the library of Giovanni Pietro Feretri of Ravenna, scholar, lawyer and bishop (d. 1557), see Fuchs (1549: 258v); noted by Caius at EtonAdv IV, 367.

71 Caius (1544b I: 299, 335, 304, 331–2), the first and last illustrated with drawings, cf. 287, and above, p. 63. Vesalius accepted these corrections in the second edition of the *Fabrica*, adapting Caius' illustration of the joint, see Figure 7.

72 This was a recent controversy. Vesalius in 1538 (Nutton 2017a: 72) says nothing about it, and makes the point only obliquely in the *Fabrica* (1543: 282). Colombo (1559: 143) was aware of the debate, criticising Galen and Vesalius for locating the origin of the straight muscles in the sternum instead of in the pubic bone. Massa (1536: 11v) was probably the first to describe the two pyramidal muscles

(although viewing them as endings of the straight muscles). At the same time, in Paris, Jacobus Sylvius (1556: 194, but published earlier) termed them 'small muscles'). Both texts are likely to have been known to Caius and antedate the traditional discoverer, Falloppia, by several years (Barcía Goyanes 1982: 367–9).

73 In Galenic anatomy purpose determined the way in which a part was created (teleology). 'Incidentally' means that this is not an intrinsic property of the individual part, but is something added or brought about later.

74 Caius first made this suggestion in his notes to Galen's *Anatomical Procedures* *(*1544: 284*)*. His first etymology is wrong, but the second is correct, see Skoda (1988: 57–8); André (1991: 203, citing Isidore for the comparison); Langslow (2000: 185, 331).

75 Francis Van Glabbeek identifies these 'two appendages' as the pyramidal muscles, small triangular muscles, found in about 80 percent of humans, which have their origin on the *linea alba* and insert onto the pubis. They have the function of tensing the *linea alba*.

76 Caius may have had experience of bell-ringing in this way in N. Italy, London, or even in Cambridge, where the largest bell in the campanile at King's weighed over two tons.

77 A criticism of Vesalius (1543: 282) and Colombo (1559: 143). Caius repeats Galen, *The Use of Parts* 5, 14: III, 393 K. and *Method of Healing* 6, 4: 10, 411 K. Modern anatomical descriptions follow Vesalius in locating the head of the muscle in the pubic bone.

78 Caius follows Galen in his argument here; modern anatomists, by contrast, see the role of the straight muscles as flexing the spine and assisting in urination, defecation and parturition.

79 Caius' argument raises a problem of identification. At first sight, he appears to be comparing the pyramidal muscles with the pronator quadratus muscle which lies deep in the forearm, comes down to the wrist and has transverse fibres. But Galen's description is not entirely accurate, as Vesalius pointed out (1543: 216/316) and, although Vesalius and Colombo (1559: 159) describe this muscle as fleshy (although not as much as others nearby), it is a muscle nonetheless. It would be odd to find Caius mistaking such an obvious muscle or confining its purpose to filling up space and providing a cushion between the two bones. A more plausible suggestion (Garrison and Hast (2014: 620, note 6) is the interosseous membrane, mentioned briefly by Galen, *Anatomical Procedures* I, 7: II, 258 K., as a membranous ligament going between the ulna and the radius. But its fibres are more oblique than transverse, and a membrane is not flesh. The fault may lie with Caius for confusing the two descriptions in the heat of the argument.

80 Galen, *Bones* 25: II, 778 K.; criticised by Colombo (1559: 143). The notion of a bone in the heart was rejected by Vesalius in the *Fabrica* (1543: 93–4), although he had followed Galen earlier in accepting this phantom, which results from the calcification of the septum in certain animals.

81 Caius used the same example, above, p. 57.

82 Although Caius uses '*fabrica*' here in its original meaning of 'forge' or 'workshop', he is also alluding to Vesalius' use of the word with a different meaning, 'make-up', in the title of his great book, *De humani corporis fabrica*. Vesalius in this copied his Paduan teacher, Giunio Paulo Grassi, who translated the title of Theophilus' Περὶ τῆς τοῦ ἀνθρώπου κατασκευῆς as *De corporis humani fabrica* (Venice: O. Scotus, 1536).

83 This is presumably a covert attack on Vesalius and his followers. Some of Vesalius' discoveries were disputed by others, e.g., Colombo (1559: 159, accusing Vesalius of 'hallucinating' over the ribs); and there was a substantial debate

between Falloppia and Vesalius (Fallopius 1561; Vesalius 1564). Other Galenists also objected that by underplaying the role of function and purpose he was missing much and describing an anatomy that was less valuable for medical practice (Skaarup 2015: 127).

84 Eusebius, *Ecclesiastical History* 2, 28, 13–14, quotes an author of about 210 describing a sect of Christians in Rome, led by Theodotus the shoemaker, who 'almost worshipped' Galen. Caius quotes the Greek of Eusebius at 1557: 36.

85 This is aimed at Vesalius, whose *De humani corporis fabrica* was written when he was in his mid-twenties (and younger than Caius). It attacked Galen, and, by implication, his own teachers, for ideas that he had himself accepted as late as 1538 (Guinter and Vesalius 1538; Nutton 2017a: 47). This 'impiety' was at least as much the cause of resentment against Vesalius as his new discoveries, many of which were eagerly accepted by other Galenists, see above, pp. 35–6.

86 Galen, *Anatomical Procedures* 2, 4: 2, 298–99 K.

87 Vesalius had been responsible for revising the Latin translations of *Anatomical Procedures, The Anatomy of Nerves* and *The Anatomy of Veins and Arteries* for the 1541–2 Giunta edition.

88 Caius (1544b: I, 335–6), argued (rightly) that Vesalius at *Anatomical Procedures* 9, 4: 2, 726 K. had misunderstood the Greek and said that the function of the septum lucidum in separating the anterior ventricles was contrary to ('not in agreement with') its name. Later editions make the correction.

89 Caius (1544b: I, 298–9). Galen, *Anatomical Procedures* 2, 11: 2, 336 K, describing the various ways in which Nature had fixed parts of the body together, compared the junction of bones in the cranial sutures to that of a '*ginglymus*', a type of buckle or hinge. Vesalius (1543: 14) had drawn it as a peg fitting into a ring, as in the fixing of an outer shutter, but Caius, correctly, drew it as a clasp-joint (see Figure. 7), backing his argument up by claiming that an English word for a hinge, 'gimmer', derived by shortening from the Greek. His argument, although perhaps not his etymology, convinced Vesalius to introduce a new, and more correct, image into the second edition of the *Fabrica* (1555: 17) alongside his original figure.

90 Caius says nothing at 1544b: I, 323–24 in his commentary on his text (195 = II, 569–71 K.), where Galen discusses the lobes. The discrepancy arose because the number of lobes varies between animals; horses have three, the pig four and the dog six or seven. The standard view, following Galen, until the publication of Vesalius' *Fabrica* (1543: 506–7) was that the human liver had five lobes; modern anatomists (and Vesalius) favour four.

91 Possibly a reference to Colombo (1559: 163), who denies their existence in humans but accepts two in birds.

92 Herophilus (about 280 BC) dissected human corpses at Alexandria in Egypt. Caius took his information from, respectively, Tertullian, *On the Soul* 10, 4 (p. 13 Waszink) and Galen, *Anatomical Procedures* 6, 8; II, 570–2 K. (= Von Staden 1989: T. 67 and 60).

93 Caius is not here referring to the text on *Anatomy* as it is printed today, and which speaks of two lobes (1, 4: 8, 536 L.; Craik 2006: 125–6), but to his own reconstruction of the lost treatise, see above, pp. 70–2. The passage is found in *The Nature of Bones* 1: 9, 168 L., but elsewhere in that tract (10: 9, 180 L.), as in *Anatomy*, the number is given as two. The number was disputed in Antiquity: Rufus believed in four or five, *Anatomy* 28: p. 175 ed. Daremberg-Ruelle, Galen in five.

94 Caius cites Tertullian, *On the Soul* 10, 4 (p. 13 Waszink = Von Staden 1989: T. 67 and 60). T

95 Galen (1551) *De anatomicis administrationibus*. Lyons: G. Rouille, a student edition, updating the version by Johann Guinter.

96 Caius 1549; Hieronymus (2005) omits this printing. Since this book finally appeared with Froben, below, note 98, this may be either a failure of memory of the part of Caius or a sign of a much earlier draft. Caius here quotes the title in Greek, although later on, above, p. 83, he uses the standard Latin form of the title, *De sanitate tuenda, The Preservation of Health*.

97 For Knolles (d. 1583), later a diplomat and MP, see Caius (1544b: II, 4); Woolfson (1998: 248–9). Presumably Caius provided him with an emended text of either the Aldine or the Basle edition in a private lesson, which Knolles then repeated for Italian students.

98 For Owen (c.1499–1588) a royal physician, see Lee and Wallis (2004). No trace of the readings of any of these MSS is found in Caius' Eton annotations. The Greek text of this tract was published in Basle by Froben, not Oporinus, in May 1548. The book finally appeared in 1549 with the original preface (Nutton 1987a: 72). Clement's manuscript was almost certainly Paris, BNF gr. 2172 (Wenkebach 1933: 208; Nutton 1987a: 58, 88), but Owen's cannot be identified for certain. It may be Leipzig, University Library gr. 50, or a series of notes and emendations by Owen, or a MS now lost (Nutton 1987a: 88–9).

99 A comparison with his other commentaries suggests that Caius in his annotations would have justified the changes that he made to the wording of the Greek text as well as any new interpretation of what the Greek meant. He may also have taken advantage of the complex debates among contemporary botanists and pharmacologists over the identification of the plants and other substances mentioned in Classical sources.

100 The second edition with the accompanying commentary (and the other books) had not been published by the time of Oporinus' death in 1568, see below, note 105.

101 Anne Bacon, née Cooke (1527/8–1610), the mother of Sir Francis Bacon, was a learned translator of works of theology from Italian and Latin that furthered the Protestant cause. She married Nicholas Bacon, Keeper of the Great Seal in 1553 (Magnusson 2004). Her sister, Lady Elizabeth Hoby (1528?–1609), was a poetess, translator and patron of musicians, and she and all her other siblings were educated in Latin, Greek, Italian and French (Priestland 2004; Lamb 2009; Crawford 2010: 38–43; Laoutaris 2010: 306–11). The comparison of these exemplary Protestants with the More family had been already made in 1550 by Roger Ascham in a letter to Jean Sturm (Crawford 2010: 39). McCallum Barry (2017: 37–43) stresses the singularity of contemporary praise of learned women, like that of Caius.

102 Mildred Cecil (1526–1589) was yet another of the Cooke sisters, and wife of William Cecil, Lord Burghley, chief minister of Queen Elizabeth (Bowden 2009; Stevenson 2009: Crawford 2010: 38–40). Margaret Clement (née Giggs) (1508–70; Wenkebach 1925: 57–60; Schoeck 1949; Bowker 2004a) was the ward of Sir Thomas More. More's daughter, Margaret, had an international reputation for her scholarship (Wenkebach 1925: 6; Reynolds 1960; Bowker 2004b; Laoutaris 2010: 298–306). Both Queen Mary and Queen Elizabeth were famous for their learning (Loades 1991: 31–4, 42–5).

103 The story of Claymond's Pliny is excellently told by Woolfson (1997). Sixteen volumes of commentary by Claymond (1468–1537) survive today in the Basle University Library and four in his old Oxford College, whose president at the time was Thomas Greenway. The Basle printer Bebel in 1531 had planned to print the commentary, and Oporinus presumably later had access to some of his

originals. Pliny's *Natural History* is the largest encyclopaedia from Antiquity and remained until the seventeenth century a major source for medicine and natural history. Caius would have heard of this famed 'missing' commentary from friends like John Clement and Edward Wotton, both fellows of Corpus in Claymond's time as president.

104 For Mounte (1496/7–1572), see MacMahon (2004). Welti (1964: 149) sees Mounte's hand behind the letter of Jociscus, below, note 106, for the return of Caius' MSS. John Gylpin may be the London merchant and traveller who came across six dubious Spaniards in 1580, and who acted as an informant for Burghley (Green 1872: 20; Lemon 1856: 503, of 1576, giving the name as George). Caius seems to have been drafted this and the following sentence a little earlier than the last one in the paragraph, which implicitly corrects it.

105 A letter of Gessner to Zwinger suggests another, and perhaps more plausible, reason (Gessner 1577: 111v). Gessner believed that Caius was sending his editions, along with the book on British dogs, to Froben and Episcopius, and that he would be asked to print them, only if they refused. He asked Zwinger to enquire if and when publication would be likely to be, knowing that Froschover already had the images of the dogs. Oporinus had been in financial difficulties for a while, and, when he sold up in 1567–8, he made special arrangements for the future printing and sale of two volumes, one of them the *Fabrica;* Caius may have thought that a similar provision had been made for these manuscripts (Steinmann 1969: 200–1).

106 Welti (1964: 148, n. 25), discusses the identity of Oporinus' heirs, among whom was, almost certainly, his nephew, Theodor Zwinger. Others sought Zwinger's help in securing the return of Caius' MSS and of the Pliny. Andreas Jociscus (fl. 1560–1570), the biographer of Oporinus, wrote from Strasbourg to Zwinger on 29 August, 1568, perhaps at Mounte's prompting (Welti 1964: 149). A year later, on 18 September, 1569, the Cambridge doctor and botanist, Thomas Penny (c. 1530–1589), perhaps at Caius' instigation, made a similar request to Zwinger: *Ne obliviscaris quaeso librorum Jo. Caij medici Angli, quos si poteris impetrare rem gratissimam illi feceris. Librorum tituli: Claymidis commentarii in totum Plinium; Jo. Caij comment. et correctiones in Galeni lib. de parva sphęra;Jo. Caij traductio et correctiones librorum Galeni de Sanitate tuenda.* ('Please don't forget the books of the English doctor John Caius; if you can get then, you will be performing a very welcome service. The book titles are: Claymond's *Commentary* on the whole of Pliny, John Caius' commentary and emendations to Galen's *Small Ball*, John Caius' translation and emendations of Galen's books on *The preservation of Health*.') I am grateful to Holger Funk for telling me about this letter (Basle University Library MS Fr. Gr. II, 19, 04).and providing me with a photograph. See also Funk (forthcoming).

107 Only Book 1 of *The Opinions of Hippocrates and Plato* was ever published, by Froben at Basle in 1549. Caius is being disingenuous about his discovery. The Greek MS on which it is based once formed part of a Laurentian MS that he saw in Florence (De Lacy 1978–1984: 31–5), but is now in the College Library, MS 47/24. How it arrived there is far from clear and may reflect very badly on Caius.

108 Galen, VII, 406–39, 440–62 K., still printing them as separate books, although Galen refers only to a single book at XIX, 108 K., identified by Boudon-MIllot (2007: 208) only with part 2.

109 Galen, VI, 836–80, VII, 1–272 K.: English translation by Johnston (2006). Caius begins his collations at EtonAdv. III, 199–248, with a similar remark about the order of the books on p. 199. His comment here is odd, for he is

clearly referring to the edition of the complete works of Galen in Greek, Basle: A. Cratander and J. Bebel, 1538 (Hieronymus 2005, no. 089), which follows the same order as that printed in the 1525 Aldine edition. But in the latter edition, part five, *Pars Quinta*, is printed with two separate paginations, with the final tract in the first half, *Dyspnea*, finishing in an elegant triangle towards the end of fol. 106r, and with the verso left blank. *The Differences between Diseases* then opens the second half on fol. 1r. Had Caius used a copy of this edition that lacked this second part, perhaps through it having been bound separately? Or was he simply careless?

110 Another book that is now lost.

111 For this position, see above, p. 13.

112 Realdo Colombo (1515–59), Vesalius' deputy and successor at Padua, mentions Caius' attendance at his dissections of female corpses (1559: 266). When Caius came to Padua, the arts lectures were held in a private house near S. Biagio, but by the time he left they had moved to the present central building, the Bo' (Caius 1574a: 184 = 147 R.)

113 Matteo Corti (1475–1544/5) had very recently moved from Bologna to Pisa as the best paid medical professor in Italy (De Ferrari 1983; Nutton 1987b). Caius (1557: *3r) says he was his one-time teacher, who encouraged him to edit *Anatomical Procedures*. He was a leading exponent of Galenic anatomy, debating some of his conclusions with Vesalius at Bologna in 1540 (Eriksson 1959). His lectures on Mondino were published posthumously in 1550 and twice after that (Corti 1550).

114 A. Cornelius Celsus, fl. 30, was the author of a Latin encyclopaedia of arts, including sections on oratory and medicine, the latter based on a substantial knowledge of learned Greek texts (Nutton 2013: 169–70). It is the most important surviving Latin medical text, and provided the Renaissance with an appropriately classical Latin medical vocabulary. None of Caius' own copies, whether in printed or manuscript form, (Grierson 1978: nos 22, 36, 108, 115) appears to have reached his College Library. For the fate of the copy he took with him, see below, Appendix I.

115 Respectively, Florence, Biblioteca Mediceo-Laurenziana, Plut73, 1; 73, 5; and 73, 6. of 1453 He did not, apparently, see two others Plut. 73, 6 and 73, 2. How Caius came to possess Gonville and Caius MS 47/24, 3, which at one point formed the opening leaves of Florence, Mediceo-Laurenziana Plut. gr. 74, 22 (De Lacy 1984: 32–3), or the fragment of *The Use of Parts* in the same Caius MS, leaves also taken from Plut. gr. 74, 22, is very unclear, and possibly discreditable (Nutton 1987a: 55–6; Berlier 2011). When it was first collated by Caius, it was intact, see EtonAdv, I, 253–99. Celsus was printed at Venice in 1524 by Lucantonio Giunta and in 1528 by the Aldine press, and at Solingen by Johann Soter in 1538 and 1540. Caius' own copy into which he inserted collations and emendations, is almost certainly that printed in Paris in 1528–29 by Wechel, see below, p. 96, note 122.

116 The first is now Vatican, Urbinas lat. 249; the others are found in Vatican, Urbinas gr. 69, 65 and 67 respectively. None of these Galen MSS is noted in EtonAdv. The suspicious Duke of Urbino was Guidubaldo II (r. 1538–1574), so his contretemps with the printer would have been quite recent.

117 Caius noted, EtonAdv II, 474, that this MS, now Vatican, Urbinas gr. 67, was not used for the Basle edition. Who the printer was is unclear: Giovanni Farri, Ricci's publisher, is a possibility, who may have borrowed it for his edition or for his revision of an earlier translation which did not appear for several years, if at all. Caius implies that he knew of another possibility; only one of the three books

remains today in the Vatican codex, but he describes it as being 'entire' when it was loaned out. Had the printer lost or failed to return the last two books?

118 For Bonamico, above, p. 89; the manuscript cannot be identified among the *recentiores* of Celsus discussed by Marx (1915: LII–LXVIII).

119 Marcellus of Bordeaux (around 350 AD) wrote a large work on drugs which included many recipes taken from the earlier writer Scribonius Largus (around 50 AD); for Celsus' use of Hippocrates, see above, note 27.

120 These manuscripts are respectively Bibliotheca Mediceo-Laurenziana Plut. 73, 1; 73, 5; and 73, 6. The former is now dated by scholars to the ninth century; the other dates are taken from colophons in the codices.

121 For these editions, see below, Appendix I. Caius was among the earliest British coin collectors, and his comments on ancient weights and measure were praised most highly by a later reader, Johann Rode (1587–1659), himself a collector. I am grateful to Andrew Burnett, whose discovery of a draft preface by an English numismatist led to me into unexpected places. Editions of Celsus from 1528 onwards, including some known to Caius, frequently contained a short poem on weights and measures by the Roman grammarian, Q. Remnius Fannius Palaemon, fl. 40 AD. Caius was providing a more scholarly and up-to-date discussion of the topic.

122 Scribonius Largus, *RecipesPreface* 13; 163, dated to 47/8 AD, although despite his citation of recipes used by members of the court, and his dedication of another book to the Emperor Claudius, it is doubtful that he ever was his personal physician. Editions of Scribonius available to Caius were published at Paris: Wechel, 1528–29, and Basle: A. Cratander, 1529. Since the former, a folio volume, also contains Celsus, it is possible that this was the volume he took with him around Italy. No commentary on Scribonius appeared before that of Rode (Rhodius) in 1655

123 Ibid., *Pref.* 14.

124 Niedermann and Liechtenhan (1968: 842–6), Sconocchia (1983: viii) and Jouanna-Bouchet (2016: CXX–CXXVI) list Marcellus's borrowings. Caius' use of Marcellus to improve an earlier author is a remarkable piece of philology, unnoticed by modern editors. Rode, a later editor of Scribonius, knew only a few emendations by Caius to the text. See Appendix I.

125 For this Galenic text, see above, p. 93, note 96.

126 An ephemeral fever, in Galenic medicine, was one that reached a crisis point every day.

127 Caius (1552; repr. in R.) A lawyer much involved in matters involving ecclesiastical property, Warmington had been a member of a commission dealing with the dissolution of monasteries under Henry VIII (Page 1911; 102; Cavill 2013: 888; and the many references in Shaw 2003), and later, as commissary to Bonner, the Marian bishop of London, in actions against evangelicals (Foxe 1563: 716). His elastic conscience allowed him to be reconciled to the Elizabethan Court and he continued to perform other legal offices (Lemon 1856: 120). He was the dedicatee of Caius' edition of *Barley Gruel* (1557: 18–19).

128 Caius (1556; repr. in R.), dedicated to Antoine Perrenot, bishop of Arras, the future Cardinal Granvelle. This more elaborate version was written in Latin for an international audience. Between 1485 and 1551 there were five devastating outbreaks of this disease in Britain and on the near Continent: its identification is far from being settled today.

129 For the first two, Caius 1556; Boudon-Millot (1999, 2007: 74–8).

130 Caius (1556): Galen, XIX, 182–221 K. He used as his base Greek text for this and for *Coma* Florence, Biblioteca Mediceo-Laurenziana, Plut. gr. 74, 3, a

thirteenth-century MS. His formulation suggests that he had not come across the second copy of this text, now Venice, Biblioteca Marciana, App. Cl. V, 4, which was at this time in the Grimani Library at S. Antonio di Castello in Venice (Westenberger 1914: XL–XLII). The treatise, however, is not by Galen, as Gadaldino recognised in his revision of Caius' version, see Galen (1565: VIII, cliii^r–clvi^r); Garofalo (2004: 313–14); its lack of authenticity was confirmed by the discovery of the genuinely Galenic treatise of the same title in Arabic translation (Lyons 1969: 75–111).

131 The text is mutilated at the beginning in both MSS, and Caius may have hoped to find yet more of it. For *Coma*, see above, p. 58.

132 Although Caius made very many notes on this book in Greek in the Eton Galen (Boudon-Millot 1999), he implies here that he knew of someone else preparing to make a new edition of the Greek. If he did, the potential edition never appeared.

133 Again, none of these annotated editions were published.

134 Caius alludes to Gadaldino and the editors of the 1565 Giuntine edition (Galen 1565: VIII, cliii^r–clvi^r), who, however, did not place it among the spurious tracts in Volume X.

135 Caius (1557). Caius inserted his corrections to *Bones* into his copy of the 1543 Paris edition, which was then sent on to Oporinus (Hieronymus (2005: 1471–6), now Basle, Frey-Grynaeus Museum, Ms I 13, nr. 19. The proposed commentary was never published. For Sir Thomas Wendy, see above, p. 8. John of Stobi, fl. 450 AD, was an anthologist, useful today particularly for works otherwise lost. Gessner had already published in 1550 a Latin translation of this summary, John of Stobi, *Anthology*, 4, 37, 14, see Jouanna (2010). Maro, '*nobilis Britannus*' (1557: 34), may be Thomas Marrow (1516–61), an MP under Mary who knew Nicholas Bacon and was involved in various land transactions with the crown (Thorpe 1982; Knighton 1998: 377), but the identification is far from certain.

136 He probably began his lectures in 1545 or 1546, and continued them for twenty years (Venn 1912: 8–9). This intervention by Henry VIII was but one of the ways in which he set out to 'modernise' his kingdom. The College of Physicians did not obtain a similar privilege until 1564, possibly at Caius' prompting (Clark 1964: 122).

137 Wendy (Caius 1557: 3–4) had been particularly interested in the Hippocratic texts on the seventh- and eight-month child. It is not clear what MS Caius used, but possibly Florence, Biblioteca Mediceo-Laurenziana, Plut. gr. 74, 3. A modern edition of the Greek fragments was made by Schoene (1932–1933) and an edition of the Arabic version, with German translation, by Walzer (1935).

138 Caius (1557: 35). Of the major MSS of *Bones*, Caius certainly collated Paris, BNF gr. 2248, and perhaps Florence, Biblioteca Mediceo-Laurenziana, Plut. gr. 74, 7. For his comments on consistency, see Caius (1544: I, 298).

139 Galen, *Bones* 11: II, 761 K. (Garofalo and Debru 2005: 67). Caius' argument is ingenious but unproven. The opening word 'this' by itself can refer only to the sacrum, and in a written text needs the heading for clarity. But if, as is likely, Galen was dictating or demonstrating, what 'this' was would be obvious to him, and the subject might then be accidentally omitted. If so, the heading would have been added soon after.

140 Caius cites *Bones* 24, 11: II, 777K. (Garofalo and Debru 2005: 83), where there is no heading. However, at the beginning of the section, 24, 1: II, 775 K. (Garofalo and Debru 2005: 81), there is found a chapter heading 'On the bones of the foot', coming between the description of the kneecap and that of the heel joint. Caius' suspicion may have been shared by the scribe of Milan, Biblioteca

Ambrosiana gr 687 (Q 87 sup), a sixteenth-century MS then still in the East, which lacks this heading.

141 Galen VI, 816–31 K. The lacuna is easily visible at Galen (1525: 2, 105r). *Pace* Hartlich (1923: LXII), arguing that Caius in 1557 used only the 1538 Basle edition, Caius' source is likely to have been Vatican, Reginensis 173, a manuscript owned by John Clement. He had earlier attempted to fill the lacuna by translating back from the Latin, probably of Donzellini's 1550 translation, although some of his retroversion is closer to that of Ricci (Nutton 1987a: 89–91). At EtonAdv II, 489, he says that Donzellini used 'a very ancient Greek MS' (probably Paris, BNF gr. 2267), and describes a Greek reading at 490, 22 as found '*in antiquo codice*', but the differences between his Eton notes and his 1557 edition are such that he must have gained access in the interim to a Greek MS which contained more than what Ricci had printed in his preface.

142 *The Opinions of Hippocrates and Plato* VI, 8, 62: V 580 K. Galen had discussed the authenticity (or not) of these 'Hippocratic' anatomical passages earlier in the same book, VI. 3, 27–31: V 528–29 K.

143 Hippocrates, *Anatomy* 8, 536–541 L...; Craik (2006).

144 *The Heart* (9, 76–93 L.; Potter 2010: 52–70) is now regarded as a much later work, probably of 280–250 BC (see Lonie 1975); *Glands* (8, 550–75 L.; Craik 2009); *The Nature of Bones* (9, 162–197 L; Potter 2010: 9–50).

145 [Hippocrates] *Nature of Man* 11: 6, 58–60 L; Galen, *Commentary on Nature of Man* II, 6: XV, 134–146 K.; Aristotle, *Investigation into Animals* 3, 2: 511^{b}24–30; 3, 3: 512^{b}2–513^{a}30: Harris (1973: 20–1, and 50–63) discusses a modern (flawed) reconstruction along the lines pioneered by Caius'.

146 [Hippocrates], *Epidemics* II, 4, 1: V, 120–26 L.

147 Galen, XIX, 13–14 K., with Boudon-Millot (2007: 138).

148 Respectively, Galen V, 580 K; IV, 537 K.; II.216 K.; Galen 1565: 286v (fragments translated into Latin by Gadaldino); and the further list of references in De Lacy (1978–1984: 672).

149 Marco Fabio Calvi of Ravenna (d. 1527) was the first translator of the 'modern' Hippocratic Corpus into Latin (1525), which appeared in print a year before the first printing in Greek (Mondrain 2017). For this tract see Calvi (1525: DC–DCI).

150 *Leverage* (4, 328–95 L; Withington 1928: 398–449) seems to summarise other related texts. The first section, headed *On the Nature of Bones*, is very closely related to that text, but is not identical with it.

151 Janus Cornarius (1500–1558) held chairs at Marburg and Jena (Mondrain 1997; Monfort 2016). A prolific translator of Greek medical and scientific texts, he knew Caius and his work. Caius is referring to his edition of translations of Hippocrates (Basle: Froben and Episcopius, 1546). For Calvi, see above, note 149.

152 No modern editor of any of these texts bothers to notice Caius' ingenious reconstruction.

153 For Gadaldino, Pastore (1998); Garofalo (2004); for Rasario, Savino (2009); for Machello, Eloy (1764: 136).

154 Rasario's translations are at best pastiches, see Garofalo (2009), and at worst based on forgeries.

155 Caius (1570b = 23–65 R.). Caius later added four entries on the fish he had seen (and eaten) in 1569–1570 (1570b 26r–29r-= 58–62 R.). See Figure 4 for Caius' addition of the English word for 'bull' to the names listed in Gessner's *Icones*.

156 Raven (1947: 49); Grigson (2016: 14–15); Funk (2017), whose appendix (345–51) provides an excellent inventory that lists when and where Gessner incorporated Caius' material into his books and his collections.

157 Egmond (2013, 2016) describes her discovery of the animal drawings in the library of the University of Amsterdam, (=ULA), MS III C 22 and 23. They supplement the plant drawings previously known from the Sammlung Trew in the Library of Erlangen University (= ERL). The surviving images of the material sent by Caius are located as follows: hartebeest, ULA MS III C 23, fol. 26; Gessner (1603: 121, but without image); the Barbary sheep, ULA MS III C 23, fol. 38; Gessner (1551–58, II: Appendix: 10), (1560a: 36); the long-tailed Arabian sheep, ULA MS III C 23, fol. 36; Gessner (1560a: 15), (1603: 773); the pod of grains of paradise, ERL, MS 2386.1: 155b verso; Jerusalem palms, ERL, MS 2386.1: 155b verso; ilex ERL, MS 2386.2: 220r (both types).

158 Caius (1570a = 3–21 R.). In its English translation (1576 = 1–47 R.) this became undoubtedly Caius' most celebrated production. Gessner (1560a: 27) knew the first version under a slightly different title: *De differentiis et moribus canum anglicorum, The Different Types and Behaviour of British Dogs*.

159 This rhetorical tour-de-force reproduces many tropes of the classical 'Consolation', see Baltussen (2013).

160 Gessner not only taught at the Carolinum, but was also a civic physician, and a leading figure in the intellectual and religious life of the city (Leu 1990, 2016a).

161 Posidippus (fl. 289 B.C.) was an influential comic writer, whose works survive today only in the form of fragments and citations. Caius took this quotation from an anthologist writing some seven centuries later, John of Stobi, *Anthology* 4, 34, 57, a work translated by Gessner (Zurich: C. Froschover, 1543: 465); an observation owed to the late Charles Brink (Brooke 1985: 58, note 18). This section, going down to 'course of life' is taken almost verbatim from Caius' Preface to *De ephemera Britannica* (1556: 116–18 = 59–60 R.).

162 Seneca, *Consolation, for Polybius* 11, 4.

163 Caius alludes to Horace, *Epistles* I, 18, 15, 'always goat's wool', a proverbial phrase for something worthless.

164 Diogenes of Sinope (404–323), the cynic philosopher, quoted by Diogenes Laertius, *Lives of the Philosophers* 6, 24, 10, said that he regarded mankind as at one and the same time the most intelligent and the silliest of all animals, to be guided by reason or, like a donkey, by a halter.

165 This sentence was not included in the 1556 preface, which also included two sentences at the end of the next sentence: For this reason, a man is accounted most fortunate for being oppressed by the smallest and fewest inconveniences of this life, a nice kind of felicity. Such is our lot, so unhappy our condition, so unfair happiness, that you may leave this life before you succeed in avoiding them.

166 Pliny, *Natural History* 26, 6, 9.

167 Plutarch, *Bringing up Children* 13:13 A.

168 The whole section is taken from Cicero, *Old Age* 23, 83–84, with slight changes. Cato the Elder (234–139 BC), Roman politician and moralist, is the leading speaker in Cicero's dialogue.

169 Socrates (469–399 BC), Athenian philosopher; Phocion (402/1–318 BC), Athenian statesman and general; Seneca (d. AD 65), Roman philosopher and writer, forced to commit suicide by the Emperor Nero; Epaminondas (d. 362), Theban general, who survived a capital trial only to die in battle; Scipio Africanus (236–183 BC), Roman general; Aristides 'the Just' (d. c. 467 BC), Athenian politician and general, ostracised in 483/2; Themistocles (c. 524–459 BC), Athenian general and politician, died in exile allegedly poisoned; Diogenes (above, n. 164), the story that he died after eating raw squid is one of several legends of his death; Aeschylus (525/4–456/5 BC), Athenian tragedian, killed when a tortoise was dropped on his head; Sophocles (d. 406 BC), Athenian tragedian; Euripides

(d. 407/6 BC) Athenian tragedian; Homer (800 BC?) epic poet, allegedly died a wandering beggar. All these deaths were famous (and in part legendary) already in Antiquity, but similar lists could be found in renaissance encyclopedias such as that of Zwinger (1565).

170 Gessner died on 13 December 1565, having contracted the plague only four or five days previously.

171 The phrase '*vivit post funera virtus*', to which this alludes, was a favourite with Caius, who had it inscribed on the tomb of Linacre in St Paul's Cathedral, as well as on his own tomb. It was a commonplace motto, see Boissard (1588: F4r p47). Its origin is extremely obscure. Angelrannus/Ingelramnus, the biographer of St Riquier, d. 1045 (*Patrologia Latina* 141 52), ended a hexameter with '*narrat post funera virtus*', which suggests that the phrase was already current.

172 This sentence, if printed correctly, forms a somewhat surprising conclusion. Caius is playing on the commonplace trope that contrasts the everlasting nature of fame with the brevity of life. The fact that Gessner has lived long enough to gain an immortal reputation is a cause for rejoicing, not for weeping as someone long compelled to remain amid the cares of this world, as the rest of the digression might suggest,

173 Terence, *The Self-tormenter*, 1.i.25

174 See above, p. 44, note 64; Funk (2016). Gessner's promise was contained in his letter to William Turner (Gessner 1562: B.8), where he mentions his own additions to Caius' original submission.

175 Caius (1570a = 1–19 R.), still containing unchanged the revised preface with its dedication to Gessner. Caius' drawings are preserved in ELA 3–5. For a later addition of the English word for bull by Caius, see Figure 4.

176 This is unlikely to have been his treatise on the pronunciation of Greek and Latin as we have it below, which makes no mention of this agreement. Gabel (1968) says nothing about this lost work, which seems to have had more to do with etymology. Both Albania/Albinia and Brutus figure in the *Histories* of John Hardyng (d. 1465) and John Rous (d. 1491), as well as in Polydore Vergil, which Caius knew well. For their antiquarian invention, see Gransden (1982: 284–6, 323–4).

177 Caius (1568), cited from the second edition (1574a, reprinted in R.; Plomer (1926–27). This is Caius' most notorious production, a vigorous attack on his Oxford counterpart, Thomas Caius (d. 1572), for suggesting in his *Assertio antiquitatis Oxoniensis academiæ* that Oxford was the senior university. John Caius published his opponent's essay along with his own. Both works are a wonderful amalgam of fact and fiction, involving such worthies as Prince Cantaber and, King Arthur, as well as the Druids as Cambridge professors brought to Rome by Julius Caesar for the edification of the Romans (Brooke (1985: 74–5); Putter (2003); Hiatt (2004); Adolph (2015); Grafton (2017); Nutton (2017b)). No one appears to have been taken in by John Caius' use of a pseudonym, 'A Londoner'.

178 Caius (1574a: 50–6 = 42–6 R.) argued on the basis of a (forged) document dated 531 and a Glastonbury charter that King Arthur had given special privileges to Cambridge. His friend Nicholas Bacon (above, p. 65) had been shown by John Croke (fl. 1534–1540), one of the six clerks in Chancery, a document in the Tower of London that mentioned privileges given by Arthur to the University of Cambridge. Caius follows John Leland (d. 1552) in rejecting the theory of John Rous that there were schools of Greek philosophy at Cricklade (a small town in Wiltshire, the name allegedly deriving from Grecolada) even before

Alfred (1574a: 150–1, 188, 208 = 120–1, 151, 167 R.), citing a (genuine) letter of Alfred about the poor state of learning in his kingdom.

179   This revision of his *Method of Healing* does not appear ever to have been printed.

180   Caius (1574c: 4 = 4 R.) dates the version as printed to 1573; Nutton (2017b) offers an appreciation, particularly of Book II. Both books developed out of Caius' Cambridge oration before Elizabeth II in 1564 (Venn 1912: 53).

181   Never published, but presumably it had been substantially completed by 1561, when Gessner referred to it as a work *On British Springs*, above, p. 32. Cf. his contemporary William Turner's *Of the Natures and Properties as well of the Bathes in England as of other Bathes in Germany and Italy*, Cologne, 1562: Arnold Birckmann; for Gessner's interest in mineral springs, see Danzi (2016).

182   Never published. It probably dealt only with ancient towns in England or the British Isles; see also above, p. 82.

183   Never published. It was written in Greek presumably as a continuation of Galen's *De libris propriis*. The great Arabic scholar Ḥunain ibn Isḥāq (809–877) also wrote a catalogue of works by Galen that were not included in his *Catalogue*, including some that were lost (Lamoreaux 2015). The Latin *Philippic History* of Pompeius Trogus, covering the history of the Graeco-Roman world down to the 20s BC, survives today only in a summary by Justin, a much later author of uncertain date.

184   Other descriptions of medical peregrinations in Italy are Gryllus (1566); Martius (1568). Caius is referring to his notes in his copy of the Aldine, EtonAdv, in which he regularly lists the owners of the MSS whose readings he quotes.

185   In this Dominican monastery, he copied variant readings for *The Use of Parts* and Galen's *Commentary on Aphorisms*, and perhaps *The Art of Medicine* from this MS (now Venice, Marcianus gr. App. Cl. V. 9), noting in his own copy of Alexander of Tralles (Caius College MS 77/44, fols. 32v, 160v, 166v and 168v) that it had once belonged to Joachim Turrianus, general of the Dominican Order, d. 1500, and that it was similar to Marcianus gr. 295. It is unclear if he saw a MS here of The *Anatomy of Muscles*, now Paris, BNF gr. 2219, which was also there at the time (Debru and Garofalo: 99), or Marcianus gr. App. Cl. V 5, another MS linked to Turrianus, which may not at this date have arrived in the library (Nutton 1979: 52–4; Jackson 2011; cf. Gārtner 2015: 91, 189). Although he knew Diego Hurtado de Mendoza (1503–1575), the Spanish ambassador to Venice and a great collector of Greek MSS (Caius 1544b: II, 3), he does not seem to have had access to his collection.

186   It did, unless Caius added the references to the other libraries later. Cardinal Bessarion left his books at his death in 1472 to the Venetian Biblioteca Marciana, although they did not fully become available for consultation until the 1520s (Nutton 1997: 23). Caius took detailed notes on Marcianus. gr, 279, 282 and possibly 275, as well as 295. Caius gained access to the Grimani library at S. Antonio di Castello through the copyist Valeriano da Forlì, EtonAdv II: A.2: *videndi copiam michi fecit literatiss. vir Valerianus de Foro Livii;* see also Lowry (1974–75). He vaguely remembered a copy of Galen's *Dyspnoea*, EtonAdv, IV, 136, 11, and noted one of *The Use of Parts* (Paris, BNF gr 2253: Nutton (1987a: 52–3); Berlier (2011)). At the Augustinian convent of S. Giovanni, he took extensive notes on a codex of Galen's larger and smaller *Method of Healing*, indicating that it had belonged to Giovanni Calfurnio, d. 1503, who bequeathed his important collection of Greek MSS to the convent. But it had apparently disappeared by 1639 (Nutton 1987a: 54, 48).

187 The first three can be identified, respectively, with Florence, Biblioteca Mediceo-Laurenziana, Plut. gr. 75.8; Plut. gr. 74.31 (or, less likely, 75.19); and Plut. gr. 74 25. The other two (probably in the same codex) have disappeared, but neither in his notes nor in his edition is there any indication of his use of a Florentine MS (Boudon-Millot 1999, 2007: 75). The book by Dioscorides is pseudonymous and not to be confused with his *Materia medica*.

188 This is now Plut. gr. 75.8, see Guardasole (2010). For Politian (1454–94), see Perosa (1980: 32), Nutton (1987a: 23–5, 32–3).

189 Given Caius' interests, it is surprising that he makes no mention here of Biblioteca Mediceo-Laurenziana, Plut. gr. 74, 7, the famous Codex Nicetas, the oldest, the most important and the most splendid of all ancient manuscripts of surgery, which contains *Bones*, whose opening words he copied into the endpaper of Vol. V of the Eton Galen.

190 Caius introduces this reminiscence to show his own learning and to confirm the antiquity and importance of the town, but his wording differs slightly, but significantly, from that of Sallust (86–35 BC). The Roman historian in his *War against Catiline*, 59–60, describes how the rebel Catiline in his last stand in 62 B.C. entrusted his left wing to someone either called Faesulanus or, more likely, from Fiesole ('*Faesulanum quendam in sinistra parte curare iubet*'), a town that had been among the earliest to go over to Catiline (24). Caius' word order suggests that he had misremembered or misunderstood what Sallust had written.

191 Given Caius' fondness for using two nouns where, in English, one would use a noun plus adjective, the two nouns should both refer to 'old Rome'. Caius compares modern Florence with the splendours of modern Rome built on visible classical ruins and recovering from the disastrous sack of 1527.

192 Caius underestimated the distance, which is roughly 4 miles, 6.6 km. Caius notes the relationship of the two towns also at 1574c: 6 = 3 R.

193 For this MS and Caius' relations with Guidubaldo II (Duke from 1538–74), see above, p. 67. Mei (2005: 135–60) gives a good overview of the history of the library, founded by Federico III, Duke from 1444 to 1482.

194 Respectively, probably Vatican, gr. 606; either gr. 610–612, 613 or 614–616; gr. 614; and probably the fragment on bandaging in gr. 876. No lexicon title corresponds to Caius' description of the lexicon, but Vatican gr. 15 is probably meant rather than the theological collections in gr. 344. For the history of the Vatican's Greek manuscripts at this period, see Devreesse (1965).

195 For Caius' use of 'book' to mean a Greek MS, see above, p. 79. Calcagnini (1479–1541) was a distinguished humanist, diplomat and teacher at Ferrara, whose literary and scientific productions enjoyed a European reputation (Marchetti et al. 1973). He translated a work on colour by the Byzantine doctor Joannes Actuarius, printed in Actuarius, *De urinis*, Paris: J. Gazeau, 1548. At his death he left his library of 1249 volumes, many of them on scientific subjects, to the monastery of S. Domenico for public consultation, and was buried beneath the door to the library. Caius will have been among the earliest visitors to examine the collection. The library at SS. Angeli, properly called S. Maria degli Angeli, was founded by Lionello d'Este in 1442, not by the more famous Ercole (Duke, 1471–1503), and received a major donation from a member of the Pico family in 1490 (Toselli 2003: 49). It was praised by a reader in 1555 for its collection of materials in Greek, Latin and Hebrew (Agnelli 1932: 45). The monastery itself was destroyed by fire in 1805, but some of its books and MSS are preserved in the Biblioteca Ariostea in Ferrara.

196 The library at San Domenico was founded in 1469 (Blume 1827: 153–5; Alce and D'Amato 1961; D'Amato 1988: 271–7, 403–5). S. Salvatore was a church

and monastery of the Canons Regular of S. Maria del Reno (Blume 1827: 160–1; Tavoni 1991). Gessner (1545: 6v) included both libraries among the five Italian collections he singled out for possessing Greek MSS.

197 The Siena library was commissioned in 1502 by Francesco Todeschini Piccolomini, Pope Pius III, to house the collection of his uncle, Aeneas Silvius Piccolomini, Pope Pius II (1405–64), but is famous more for its illuminated MSS and its frescoes than for its classical MSS.

198 The origins of Siena go back to the Etruscans long before Brennus. Whether the name comes from a local Etruscan tribe, Saena, or via the Gallic tribe Senones, is far from clear. If the latter, there may well be the etymological connection suggested by Caius. Pomponius Mela, *Chorography* 3, 48, 1 describes a Sena *'in britannico mari,'* i.e. the island of Sein in the sea off Brittany. Caius misunderstands the adjective as referring to Britain. Brennus, chief of the Senones who sacked Rome in 390 BC, was transformed by Geoffrey of Monmouth *History of the Kings of England*, 3, 1–10, into a Brennius, King of Northumberland, who first married the daughter of the King of Norway and later the heiress of the Duke of the Allobroges. With his brother Belinus Brennus led the Gauls against Rome, capturing the city and tyrannically ruling it until his death. Caius in a note in his copy of Polydore Vergil, Gonville and Caius Library, F. 3. 10, p. 24, criticises Vergil for not realising that Brennus had invaded England

199 Caius' memory or handwriting may be at fault, for the 1589 catalogue mentions no MS of Pliny at S. Maria. But at S. Marco there was a magnificent Pliny (MS 791–2, now Biblioteca Mediceo-Laurenziana, Plut. 82, 1–2), as well as a textually much more important older MS (MS 793, now Florence, Biblioteca Riccardiana 48). The Bologna Esdras (in reality, a Hebrew scroll of the Pentateuch) was regarded as so ancient that it was kept with the relics of St Dominic. By the nineteenth century it had been identified as a much later thirteenth-century manuscript, but was still thought sufficiently valuable to be removed by Napoleon to Paris, from which it was returned, damaged, to the library of the Archiginnasio in 1815, now Cod. Ebr. 1 (Blume 1827: 146; Modona 1889: 323–4; Alce and D'Amato 1961: 79).

200 The university of Pisa, founded in 1343, was effectively closed in 1526, but revived again with new students in 1543 (Schmitt 1974, 1989: ch. IX; Grendler 2002: 74–7; Davies 2009: 81–99).

201 For Corti, see above, p. 14; Francesco Gallo da Pontremoli taught medicine at Pisa (Davies 2009: 215–18); Antonio Musa Brasavola (1500–55) was professor of medicine at Ferrara (Gliozzi 1972); Ippolito (d. 1558) and Giambattista Canano (1515–79), sons of an earlier Giambattista (d. 1550), both held chairs at Ferrara (Gliozzi 1974). The younger Giambattista was particularly famous as an anatomist (O'Malley 1964: 440). Unless Caius has mistaken the Christian name, Niccolò Bonaccioli is probably the son of Luigi Bonaccioli, a Ferrarese doctor and writer on gynaecology active in the 1520s and 1530s. Grendler (2002: 101–6) gives a succinct history of the university of Ferrara.

202 Probably Alessandro Guarino, who taught Latin and Greek at the University from 1505 to 1556 (Borsetti 1735: II, 107–9; Franceschini 1970: passim; Cerroni 2003); Marco Antonio Antimaco (1473–1552) was a famous translator from the Greek who opened his own school at Ferrara to teach Greek before becoming professor at the university (Borsetti 1735: II, 144; Franceschini 1970: 31–64). The immediate controversy over the pronunciation and spelling of Greek and Latin was inaugurated by Erasmus in his *De recta latini graecique sermonis pronunciatione* (Basle: Froben, 1528), a valiant attempt by the leading humanist to introduce order into a multiplicity of local pronunciations across

Europe. In 1535 John Cheke and Thomas Smith, both well known to Caius, see above, pp. 27, 7, introduced the reformed pronunciation of Greek into Cambridge (Cheke 1555; Smith 1568a). In 1542, the Chancellor, Stephen Gardiner, banned the reformed pronunciation of both languages, but, despite his authority, it continued to exist. Caius also took aim at two new theories of a reformed English spelling, one by Smith (1568b), and the second, in part dependent on it, by John Hart (1569).

203   For another memory of the Greek churches in Venice, see Caius (1570b: 5 = 30 R).

204   For Bonamico, above p. 89, and for Caius' collations of his MS of *The Use of Parts*, now Paris, BNF gr. 2281, see Berlier (2011); Bocchi (1488–1562), was a classical scholar and translator at Bologna (Rotondò 1969); Pompilio Amaseo (*sic*) (1513–86) was a Bolognese humanist who became professor of Greek (Avesani 1960); Egnazio (1478–1553) was a celebrated teacher of Latin in Venice, and well acquainted with Greek also (Mioni 1981).

205   This was a traditional formulation for the medieval Studium Urbis and the Studium Curiae. But they had long been amalgamated, and the university itself had been completely reorganised after the 1527 sack of Rome (Andretta 2011: 352–66). It is possible, however, that Caius meant to refer to both the university and the Collegio Capranica, which (1574c: 184 = 147 R.) he says was sometimes called the Sapienza Capranica.

206   While Caius almost certainly knew Münster in Basle, it is unclear if he ever met the others personally, see above, p. 19. Melanchthon (1497–1560), professor at Wittenberg, and the leading educator in Germany, was particularly interested in anatomy (Helm 2001). Camerarius (1500–74), a notable Greek scholar and one of the editors of the 1538 Basle edition of Galen, was professor at Tübingen from 1535 to 1541, when he moved to Leipzig (Baron 1978). Münster (1488–1552) was a Hebraist and cartographer, who taught in Basle from 1529 until his death (Priesner 1997). Drivère (c.1504–1554) studied and practised medicine at Louvain, although he did not obtain the chair of medicine there until 1542 (which might suggest that Caius met him on his return from Italy). For his career and his role in the famous blood-letting controversy (O'Malley 1964: 66–9, 429).

207   For the wider context see Waquet (2001: 160–7). The problems with the spelling and pronunciation of all three languages remain unresolved to this day. Erasmus spent the years 1510–1515 in Cambridge as Professor of Divinity (Caius 1574a: 21–2 = 19–20 R). Caius knew the printer Froben in Basle and published two of his editions (1544, 1549) with him. Levinus may be Erasmus' friend Ammonius Levinus (1488–1557), who from 1541 to 1544 was living as a Carthusian monk near Brussels (Allen 1906–1958: V, 487), but a more likely candidate is Levinus Lemnius (1505–1568), a Dutch physician who had studied at Louvain before coming to Padua, where he attended Vesalius' lectures (O'Malley 1964: 136). He shared an interest in the natural world with Caius.

208   Caius (1574d = 3–19 R.); English translation, with notes, by Gabel (1968), who dates its composition to late 1569 or early 1570, although part could well have been written earlier. Caius, as might be expected, insisted in his college statutes on the old pronunciation.

209   A long sentence, mainly in asyndeton, different in style to anything else in this book, and perhaps a sign that this part was never completed to Caius' satisfaction, cf.above, p. 30. Very few of the words found here are used in the tract on pronunciation itself, and at least one is given an apparently different meaning. 'Scotism' in the tract (9–10) refers to the Scots' method of pronunciation, here

it is joined with 'logic-chopping' as if in its customary meaning of a generally derided medieval philosophy derived from Duns Scotus (c. 1266–1308).

210 For which his collations in Eton (Figure 9) and Cambridge provided the base. He seems not to have collated manuscripts for many treatises, some of them substantial, but he made emendations to all of them with the exception of three (minor) tracts. The list is given in Nutton (1987a: 109–10.

211 A point made at length in 1544b: pref. 2.

212 Cf. above, p. 73. It is not clear which editor or translator Caius is alluding to, possibly Rasario, whose Greek sources for the Latin versions of Hippocratic commentaries were not published in his lifetime. Modern research has shown that many of them are at best pastiches, see above, p. 98, note 154 .

213 Durling (1961) is fundamental for publication details. Greek and bi-lingual editions were always extremely rare. Caius' plea, very opportune in the 1550s, was by 1570 outdated. Galenic translations and editions declined substantially and rapidly in numbers from 1560, as newer authors and, to a certain extent, Hippocrates replaced the smaller texts of Galen. The later Giuntine complete editions seem to be old stock reissued with a newly dated title page.

214 E.g. Seneca's *Letters to Lucilius* and Plutarch's *Consolation, for Apollonius*. Caius is also alluding to Galen's comments on titles in *My own Books*, pref. 12:XIX, 11 K.= Boudon-Millot (2007: 136). Many ancient writings, including many by Galen, have a title in the form of the topic, followed by the name of a dedicatee. Caius is perhaps taking aim at his contemporaries' liking for fanciful titles, e.g. Sir Thomas Elyot's *The Castell of Helth*, London: T. Bethelet, 1541, and, in particular, Paracelsians, with obscure titles such as *Paragranum* and *Philosophiae ad Athenienses*. He may have forgotten that Gessner's most famous work on medicine was his *Thesaurus Euonymi philiatri (The Treasury of Euonymus, friend of physicians)*, Zurich: A. Gessner and L and R. Wyssenbach, 1552 (and in various translations).

215 For this and the following entry, see Appendix I.

216 'Castigare' and its cognates are used by Caius to indicate some textual editing, involving emendation and, often, a choice between variant readings. Ricci and Gadaldino in their editions of the Latin Galen regularly place alternative readings in the margins, and Robert.Constantin in his edition of Celsus (Lyons 1566: J. Tournaesius), even included longer notes there. A later annotator of the Wellcome copy of Constantin's edition, EPB 1402, added further variants from at least four MSS. Caius' collations and suggested emendations for the texts that were not eventually published are preserved in CULAdv and, much more substantially, in EtonAdv. (Fig. 7). The extent of his interventions varies considerably from treatise to treatise, and involved checking earlier Latin translations as well as Greek MSS and the annotations of others, see Nutton (1987a) for a detailed account of the volumes. The great majority were not published, and would have required considerable transcription to reach a publishable state.

217 Only Book VII, 8–14 (= III, 394–581 K.) was printed.

218 Although he did not know it, Caius was anticipated by Ricci in 1544, see above, p. 98, note 141.

Appendix I

The lost writings of John Caius

Save for the volumes seen through the press by Archbishop Parker, his literary executor, and, in the twentieth century, the *Annals* of his college and of the College of Physicians, none of the works mentioned in his *Autobibliography* as still unpublished ever appeared in print. But traces of some of them remain. In an annotation in his copy of Gessner's *Icones*, he remarked that he had noted in his book on *The Agreement of the British vocabulary with Greek and Latin* the coincidence of the word for crab with the Greek καραβος.[1] His treatise on *The Ancient Towns of Britain*, which contained a summary of his *History of Norwich*, will also have included discussions about the origin of the names of the towns along the lines briefly indicated here, cf. above, p. 86, note 25, and in *The Antiquity of Cambridge University*.[2] Similarly, had he lived, he would undoubtedly have passed on to his printers many of his conjectures and some at least of the many readings of Greek manuscripts of Galen he had seen in England and Italy and transcribed into the margins of his copy of the 1538 Basle edition of the Greek Galen, now at Eton.[3] His notes on *Anatomical Procedures* were later copied out by Lancelot Browne (c. 1545–1605), a royal physician, more famous as the father-in-law of William Harvey.[4] Another fellow of the College of Physicians, Theodore Goulston (1572–1632), also transferred many of Caius' suggestions into his own volume of the Basle Galen, some of which he later used in his own edition of some Galenic works.[5] It was the identification of Goulston's volumes in the Marsh Library Dublin that first drew attention to Caius' notes, and led to significant investigations into the Eton volumes and into John Clement's Aldine edition of Galen that Caius drew upon.[6]

Little, however, was known about Caius' work on Latin medical authors, and especially his work on two Latin medical writers, Cornelius Celsus and Scribonius Largus, despite his comments in his *Autobibliography*, above, p. 68. He had taken a printed edition of Celsus with him on his travels around Italy, comparing its text not only with two other printed editions but also with three manuscripts from Florence, one from Urbino and one from Padua. From them, as well as from others he collated later in England, he constructed his own edition, also emending the text on the basis of parallels in Hippocratic texts. Having completed his work on Celsus, he turned to another Latin author, the pharmacologist Scribonius Largus.[7] In the absence of manuscripts, he emended Largus' drug book with the aid of citations he found in the fourth-century writer Marcellus of Bordeaux. He claims to have provided commentaries or notes to both authors, although, as we shall see, this may not be entirely true. Even if he had set out to edit them separately, he later decided to publish them together, preceded by a preface dealing with the style and argument of Celsus, the weights and measures used by Celsus and Scribonius, and the true character and design of the Roman denarius, which he illustrated from a silver denarius in his own collection. The whole volume was completed by a detailed index, above, p. 68. Although these editions were almost finished by the early 1550s, they had still not been sent to the printer when Caius wrote his *Autobibliography*. His London inventory shows that Caius owned at least four copies of Celsus, none of which remains in his college library, but it makes no mention of any Scribonius.[8] This silence need not mean that by 1573 he already sent both editions off to press, for at least one printing of Celsus also contained a text of Scribonius that could easily have been overlooked by the maker of the probate inventory.

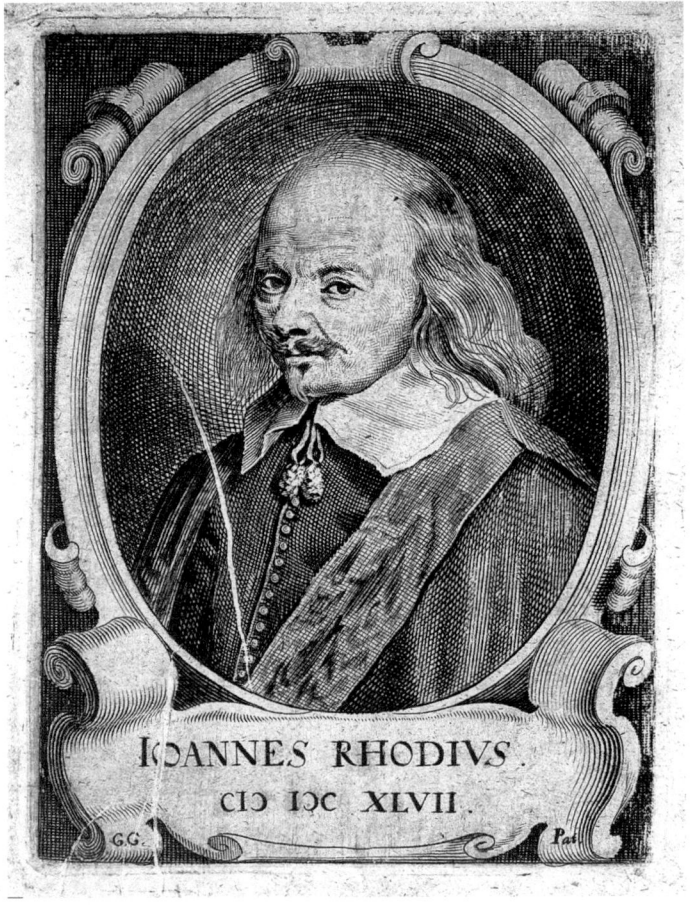

Figure 10 Johann Rode (1587–1659), *De acia dissertatio*, Copenhagen: 1672. Frontispiece.
Copyright Wellcome Collection.

Although neither of Caius' editions can be identified today and must be presumed lost, traces remain of them in the writings of a later owner, the Danish physician and scholar Johann Rode (Rhodius). Rode (1587–1659) had studied at Wittenberg, Marburg, Basle and Copenhagen, before moving to Padua, where he became the superintendent of the university botanical garden in 1631. It was a post he swiftly gave up 'for domestic reasons', but he remained in Padua as a physician, allowing foreign visitors and students to have access to his remarkable collection of coins and manuscripts in Latin and Greek.[9] Rode, an excellent Latinist, had planned to publish the whole corpus of ancient Latin medical texts, and particularly Celsus, even before his departure for Italy in 1621. He discussed his intentions with the celebrated Danish scholar and antiquarian Ole Worm (1588–1654), and it was Worm who persuaded the Danish Chancellor, Kristian Friis of Kragerup (1581–1639), to pass on a copy of Celsus to Rode to take with him.[10] Friis was a central figure in the intellectual life of Denmark, sponsoring many young Danes, including Rode himself, to travel and study elsewhere in Europe.[11] It is not clear from Worm's letter whether Friis, the possessor of a substantial library, had had the volume in his possession for some time, and had earlier loaned it to another scholar or was merely an intermediary in obtaining it from this individual, whom Worm does not name and of whose intellectual abilities he had no high opinion. How or when the book arrived in Denmark remains unclear. At this stage Worm appears not to have known the identity of the annotator, save that he was a learned man, although either he or Rode soon discovered that it was Caius.[12]

Once in Padua, the volume was proudly shown off to visitors. In 1639 Rode's friend, Giacomo Filippo Tomasini, recorded it in his catalogue of manuscripts in Paduan libraries, describing it as containing 'emendations (*castigationes*) of the Briton John Caius to Celsus'.[13] He also noted there a manuscript of Celsus 'in no way inferior to any others' in Rode's library, but made no mention of Scribonius Largus or of the prefatory material.

Tomasini's description of manuscripts in Paduan libraries, although still valuable, is far from accurate, as can be seen from an Oxford scholar's reminiscences of his visit to Rode's collection. The English doctor and traveller John Greaves arrived in Padua in November 1635, staying there for several months. A decade or so later, he began an important work on numismatics, in which he tried to establish the relationship between the weights and measures of the ancients and those of his own day, and particularly the denarius.[14] This was something that, in his view, had been either completely neglected or treated superficially, except by two scholars, the Frenchman Nicolas-Claude Fabri de Peiresc (1580–1637) and John Caius. Greaves vaguely remembered that Caius had written a special study of the Roman denarius as part of the preface to his edition of Celsus, illustrated with a drawing of a coin from his own collection, but confessed that he did not know what had become of the tract. However, he knew that Caius' copy of Celsus, 'wth many variae lectiones out of ye best MSS is in ye hands of Rhodius a Dane, who promised me att Padua to publish it, & I hope will performe it.'[15] This was not the first time that Greaves had mentioned this volume and his visit to Rode, for in a marginal note in an Almanac of 1637, but probably not entered until 1639–40, he had described four items '(to be?) edited by the scholarly Rode' (*Rhodii arte emenda(nda/ta?)*): Caius' notes on Celsus, a preface on the style and argument of Celsus along with a true explanation of the denarius; and Pomponius Largus, emended in Italy.[16] This entry confirms that the volume in Rode's library contained material on both authors, as well as the prefatory matter, rather than simply notes on Celsus.

The information provided by Worm, Tomasini and Greaves also makes it clear that what they saw was not a manuscript of Celsus but a single volume with collations and emendations that began with Celsus and ended with Scribonius Largus, and that included the prefatory matter. This was almost certainly Caius' annotated copy of Celsus that he took round Italy, and into which he would have later tipped the two discursive sections. The 1529 edition of Celsus (Paris: S. Silvius for C. Wechel), which also contains the *editio princeps* of Largus, has enough room for manuscript collations such as Caius entered into the Eton Galen, and the phrase used by both Greaves and Rode 'emended in Italy' would fit precisely what Caius says of his activities there in his *Autobibliography*.[17] This identification would also explain Rode's perplexity about the absence of almost any indication of Caius' work on Largus, known to him from the *Autobibliography*, for no manuscripts of Largus were available in Italy, and his commentary appears to postdate his return to England. Had Caius died, Rode wondered, before he could complete the edition, or was there another volume that is now lost?[18] If Caius had in fact made notes on Largus, as he implies, of the kind he appended to Galen's *Anatomical Procedures*, Rode's book is unlikely to have been that edition, and he would have used the quotations in Marcellus elsewhere to improve the text. But it is also possible that Caius never got round to writing down his insights or the notes that he planned, and that his comments in his *Autobibliography* relate to his work on Celsus.

Rode was well aware of the importance of Caius' notes. In the preface to his edition of Scribonius Largus, he expressed his thanks to Friis for his kindness in passing on this remarkable book. It contained many conjectures to the text of Celsus that 'brilliantly elucidated the text, and which reveal Caius' genius at solving textual difficulties that have defeated others through his outstanding knowledge of ancient literature'.[19] Rode may well have been inspired by Caius' examples to write his own study of *Weights and Measures* and a *Life of Celsus*, both published by Thomas Bartholin as a sort of Appendix to the revised version of Rode's *De acia*.[20] But the one reference made by Rode to Caius in them, on the date of Celsus, p. 44, is more likely to be taken from the *Autobibliography*, and both of his dissertations contain much material from later writers.

Although Rode says almost nothing about Caius' work on Largus, he does, however, cite him several times for emendations of Celsus both in his own edition of Largus and in his earlier study of ancient suturing, *De acia*. So, for instance, in the commentary on Largus, *Comp. 53*: p. 33,8 ed. Sconocchia, he remarks that Caius had replaced all the instances of '*forceps*' in Celsus with '*forfex*', which is found in the early editions of Scribonius, a change that was accepted by Friedrich Marx in his edition of Celsus (1915: 457) and by more recent editors. A few pages later, he credits Caius with correcting the vulgate παροντίδας to παρυλίδας in Celsus, VI, 13, 4, on the basis of the parallel in Largus (*Comp. 61*: p. 36,11 ed. Sconocchia). Elsewhere he commends Caius for emendations that have been accepted by modern editors on the basis of good manuscript readings, some of which Caius may already have found during his examination of Florentine manuscripts, above, p. 68. At Celsus VI, 9,6 = p. 284,6 ed. Marx, Rode accepts the reading *isque per testas excidet,* on the basis of MSS in Milan and Venice, noting that Caius had already approved of it: *auctoritate codicis Ambrosiani, Divi Antonii Venetiis et Rhodii. quod etiam Caius probauit*. At Celsus II, 33 = p. 98,1 ed. Marx, Rode follows Caius in reading '*tamarix*', citing in support a Venetian codex. Similarly, at Celsus III, 21, 10 = p. 133,9 ed. Marx, he justifies his and Caius' reading: *& scilla cocta delingitur,* as a reading he had found in the best of the Florentine codices, which Caius had also collated earlier. At Celsus V, 26, 23 D = p. 221,21 ed. Marx, Caius is praised for retaining the MS reading '*transuit*', when others wished to change it, although Rode wondered what he might have written, had he wished to emend. Finally, in two places, Celsus, VII, 4 and VIII, 10,1H = p. 391,4 ed. Marx, he accepts Caius' reading '*vinctura*' in place of the vulgate '*iunctura*', a correction demanded by the sense of the passage as well as by the authority of the oldest Florentine manuscript.[21] All these changes can be found in modern editions, although ascribed there to manuscripts rather than to Caius' ingenuity. No wonder then that Rode valued the work of his predecessor so highly, and was disappointed to find so little that he could use in his edition of Scribonius.

Rode's plans for an edition of ancient Latin medical texts soon became known across Europe, and scholars in Italy and elsewhere eagerly provided him with information on their own and others' manuscripts. It was a huge task, like rolling a stone up a hill, as Thomas Bartholin remarked in a poem of encouragement, but for Rode, as for Sisyphus, the task proved unending.[22] He was always on the point of publishing, and constantly promising to do so.[23] From at least 1637 until he died, Worm's letters are filled with requests to Rode to publish and to Danes in Padua to find out exactly what was going on.[24] His relative Thomas Fuiren reported back in 1639 that the Scribonius was almost finished and that Rode had stopped working on his Celsus, since all that remained was to produce a fair copy for the press.[25] But it was a further sixteen years before the edition of Scribonius appeared, although Rode had already sent at least a copy, and possibly his original, of the Largus to Worm in 1653. Worm's letter of that year to another relative,

Willem Worm, in Padua implies that the Celsus was also now finished, and that the young man should be able to bring it or a copy back to Denmark on his return.[26]

Rode was a difficult man to deal with. Despite many attempts to lure him back to Denmark, he remained in Padua, preferring, according to Otto Sperling, who knew him in his later years, to live in poverty rather than give up his independence.[27] Many of his books, however, did return, being inherited by his widow's brother-in-law, Thomas Bang (1600–1661), professor of Greek at Copenhagen and University Librarian. It was he who passed on Rode's edition of Celsus, along with all the other relevant material, to Rode's friend, the great Danish anatomist, Thomas Bartholin (1616–80), who undertook to revise it for the press.[28] The promised edition, when it arrived, proved a great disappointment when compared with the abundance of learning displayed in the edition of Scribonius and in the *De acia*. It contained little more than a substantial number of variant manuscript readings in a somewhat confused and undigested state.[29] Bartholin set to work to provide a proper commentary on Celsus, but he had only reached the end of Book V, when in 1670 fire destroyed his family mansion at Hegested, along with most of his library. As he wittily wrote, *abiit . . . noster Celsus ad excelsos*.[30] This was a great loss, for he had little opportunity to repeat Rode's collations of all the manuscripts of Celsus and other ancient writers. Nothing further is heard of Caius' *Castigationes*, which must be presumed to have been burnt along with Rode's papers, thus depriving scholars of an opportunity to assess Caius'expertise in Latin authors.

Notes

1 Gonville and Caius College Library, L.19.4, p. 212.
2 Caius (1574a: 48–50 = 40–1 R.).
3 Nutton (1987a).
4 London, British Library, classmark 540 e 8.
5 Dublin, Marsh Library, classmark P. 3.2, 18–22; Kozluk (2010)
6 Gundert (2006); Gärtner (2015: 190).
7 The manuscript used for the *editio princeps* of 1528 is now lost, and no other manuscript was known until Sergio Sconocchia's discovery of the Toletanus in 1974 (Sconocchia 1983: IX; Jouanna-Bouchet 2016: CXIII–CXX).
8 Grierson (1978: nos 22, 36, 108, 115). To judge from the prices, the first two may have been folio editions, one marked as 'old'.
9 Tomasini (1654; 98, 305); Hoffmann (1856); Bruun (1893); Ducceschi (1929–30: 319–20, summarising letters in Rome, Biblioteca Lancisiana, Ms V.13); Snorrason (1965, but adding little to Bruun); Mariani (1995); Grell (2017: 144–6).
10 Bruun (1893: 67); Worm (1751: I, 59–60, dated 28 Feb., 1621).
11 Bruun (1893: 25–8).
12 Worm (1751: I, 60, dated 28 Feb., 1621): *apud alium, hisce, ut nosti, imparem latitabat*. In the following undated letter-(1751: I, 60–1) he advised Rode to look at the second volume of the *De piscibus* of Gessner, dedicated to Caius,

especially his contributions towards the end of the second volume, '*quo ad eius commendationem haud parum faciet.*'

13 Tomasini (1639: 138). For the relations of Rode with Tomasini, see Bruun (1893: 44–51, 146–8), Snorrason (1965: 53–4).

14 For Greaves, see Maddison (2004), ODNB 486–87; Shalev (2005).

15 Oxford, Bodleian Library, Add MS C 299, f.114: neither Greaves nor this section of this miscellaneous manuscript is mentioned in Madan's catalogue (1905: V, 305–6, no. 27613). I am grateful to Andrew Burnett for this information and for a photograph of the entry, which he considers to be part of an unpublished preface to Greaves' *On the Roman Foot and Denarius*, published in 1647.

16 *Jo. Caii comm. In Celsum. Praefatio de stylo et argumento Celsi; De ponderibus et mensuris, item de vera denarii ratione; Pomponius Largus in Italia emendatus. Rhodii arte emenda(nda/ta?)* Shalev (2005: 83, note 26: 84, pl. 1, showing the entry), rightly suggests that Pomponius is a mistake for Scribonius.

17 This is likely to have been the volume numbered 36 in Grierson's list of Caius' books (1978: 515), which is valued higher than other copies of Celsus.

18 Rhodius (1655: sig. B 2r): *Quod vero de Libris propriis memorat Johannes Caius in emendando Largo institutum vel interrupit fatum, vel cura posteritatis minor euertit.*

19 Rhodius (1655: sig. B 1r*): Nec [Frisius] verbis id tantum prolixe testatus magnae sibi curae, verum libro etiam Ioannis Caii Britanni diligentia olim in Italia emendato e literarum supellectili sua óptimis cuiuscunque generis autoribus refertissima benigne comitatum dimisit*; sig. B 2r: *Unum igitur ab ingenio praesidium restabat, cui artificiosa coniectura tot difficultates eluctari integrum videbatur. Conatui accessit genius in hoce literarum genus procliuis qui non mediocri priscorum librorum usu iam diu perceperat varias tot errorum causas, quibus plerique turpiter scatent.*

20 Bartholin, preface to Rhodius (1672: sig. B 1r–2v).

21 The first reference cannot be found, but Rode may have meant to cite VII, 20, 1 = p. 340, 24 ed. Marx, rather than VIII, 8, 1, A or VIII, 22, 2 = pp. 385, 23 and 409, 4 ed. Marx. The emendations are found respectively in Rhodius (1655: 93r; 121r, 453r, 201r, 291r; 1672: 143, 160, 161–2).

22 Bruun (1893: 68–9).

23 Not all the delay was his fault, as he kept constantly searching for, and finding, new manuscripts to collate, see his letters to Heinsius in Burmann (1727: 445–51, 457). Gabriel Naudé (1667: 405) in a letter of March 1636, sympathised that the collation of Vatican MSS was delaying the project.

24 Worm (1751: I, 68 (1637), *quid Celsus noster? An in carceres damnatus?*; I, 554, dated 8 Sept. 1639: *sed ecquando integrum Celsum tantopere expectatum?*; I, 560, dated 8 Sept. 1639 (to Henrik Fuiren); I, 71 (1640); I, 73 (March, 1641); I, 94 (1650); II, 122, dated 17 Dec. 1553 (to Willem Worm).

25 Worm (1751: I, 556, dated 1 Dec. 1639, from Henrik Fuiren): *Cornelius Celsus vero ejus opera repurgatus jam quiescit, nihil fereque ad ejus impressionem desideratur quam ut nitide describatur.*

26 Worm (1751: II, 1122, dated 17 Dec. 1653 (to Willem Worm): *Cum Patavium perveneris, Celsum habebis egregiis notis a Rhodii illustratum. Nuper specimen transmisit Scribonii*).

27 Wuttke (1974: LXXVII–VIII): *Hance ego Stoicam philosophiam uti admiror, ita non intelligo.*

28 Bartholin (1667a: 307–8), *Ep.* 83, a letter of 7 September 1662 to Jacob Horst; (1667b: 208–9), *Ep.* 34, a letter of 18 October 1662 to Guy Patin: *De Cornelio*

Celso Rhodii nostri qvid sperandum sit, indicabo. Suppellex viri beati transiit in possessionem Thomae Bangii, Affinis illius, Academiae nostrae Professoris meritissimi, qui mihi tradidit & concredidit quicqvid inter reculas ejus inveniri potuit ad Celsum spectans. Presumably Caius' *Castigationes* was included among the other items of relevance.

29 Bartholin (1667b: 209): *Habeo igitur Rhodii Varias lectiones, ejusdem Notulas & Lexicon pene absolutum. Promisi me in ordinem cuncta reducturum, ubi per ocium licuerit, ne tanto thesauro & indefesso labore privetur Respubl. Literaria. Sed magno mihi labore stabit, qvum confusa pleraque sunt scripta. Possideo & eiusdem Rhodii Varias Lectiones, Notas et Lexicon in Vegetium Mulomedicum.*

30 Bartholin (1670: 58) = O'Malley (1961: 22).

Appendix II

John Caius and religion in early Elizabethan Cambridge

The ransacking of Caius' rooms on 13 December 1572 is a dramatic episode in the history of Elizabethan Cambridge. An anonymous letter, undated, but almost certainly written earlier in the year, denounced the 'preposterous government of Dr Caius', accusing him of maintaining within his college 'copes, vestments, albs, tunicles, censers, crosses, tapers, also all kinds of mass books, porteses, pyxes, grails, with all massing abominations and termeth them the college treasure.' He was accused of forbidding the Fellows to talk about his retention of these things, as well as of setting up a crucifix and other idols. He was alleged to have refused to examine students in their religious beliefs, as happened in other colleges, and to have discouraged them from attending the university sermon. The complaint ends with examples of the Master's delinquent theology, especially his belief in the value of good works.[1] Equally significant in the eyes of the author or authors was Caius' tyrannical behaviour as Master, although, sandwiched between accusations of antipathy to the 'true religion', this may not have attracted much notice from the cleric to whom they were addressed. This was almost certainly Edwin Sandys, bishop of London, for it was he who wrote 'very earnestly' to the vice-chancellor, Dr Byng, on the matter. Aided by two of Caius' neighbours, Dr Whitgift, the Master of Trinity, and Dr Goade, the Provost of King's, Byng obtained an inventory of the 'treasure', or, as he put it in a letter to the chancellor, William Cecil, Lord Burghley, 'much popish trumpery'. There followed a raid on Caius' rooms, burning and smashing whatever they could find in three hours of mayhem, fuelled by a religious fervour that would brook no moderation. Soon after, Caius withdrew to his London house, sick in both body and mind.

This episode raises two separate but related issues. What evidence do we have for Caius' religious beliefs other than the condemnations of his accusers, for whom true Christianity depended on faith alone? and, second, how does it relate to the wider religious changes in Cambridge in the 1560s and early 1570s? Caius' misfortune, it is argued, was the result not only of his conservatism, but also of the growing dominance of evangelicals in Cambridge, not least after the papal excommunication of Queen Elizabeth and the incitement of those still loyal to Rome to cast off their allegiance to the queen. Sympathy for anything that might smack of Rome could therefore be viewed as something more serious than an individual foible, and exacerbate local tensions within a college.

Defining the religious position of John Caius is not easy. That he was out of sympathy with the growth of evangelical Christianity is not in doubt. He disliked this 'new religion' that was pullulating everywhere, and desecrating the churches of his youth.[2] A confessed conservative in everything, and unwilling to change unless it was absolutely necessary, he saw little wrong in espousing positions that others would have thought dangerous. Whether through insouciance or a desire to tweak the noses of his opponents, he included in his *History of Cambridge University* details and documents that would in some circles have raised eyebrows at least.[3] The first document cited at length is a letter of 1554 from Philip II thanking the university for its loyal sentiments towards him on his entry into his new kingdom. Not only is the monarch given the full title of king of the Spains and described by Caius as 'Most illustrious King', but the point that Caius wishes to prove by quoting the letter verbatim is not immediately obvious.[4] A similarly unnecessary reference to Philip occurs when he describes his own college as retaining the name of Gonville Hall 'until the time of Philip and Mary, rulers of England'.[5] The select list of distinguished clerical Chancellors in Caius' lifetime mentions John Fisher, Stephen Gardiner and Reginald Pole, who is given his full title of cardinal of the Holy Church and archbishop of Canterbury.[6] Edward, Lord North, who retired from political life under Elizabeth, is described as a man 'of notable piety' and cited as a famous alumnus of Pembroke alongside Thomas Lupset, the translator of Chrysostom as well as a Galen editor.[7] By contrast, a relatively minor change in the regulations for disputations under Edward VI is preceded by a parenthesis declaring disapprovingly that in his reign 'innovation began to take over everything'.[8] The repetition in the work's preface of the standard trope that history is more than an account of past deeds but should also be a guide to prudent and wise conduct in the future could appear to one who has read to the end of the book a manifesto for a return, not just to a pre-Edwardian Catholicism, but even to papal jurisdiction. None of the Catholic references detected in the text need be interpreted in that light, for Caius was quoting the official titles at the time, but cumulatively they indicate a definite anti-evangelical standpoint.

Caius also had many Catholic friends, most notably John Clement, who had served in the household of Thomas More and whose family kept alive the memory of More (and much else) in their long exile in Malines.[9] The London College of Physicians, over which he often presided, was also viewed as a nest of papists, not least because it was far easier for medical graduates of Padua to enter than for most London practitioners. Several Fellows of the college fled abroad during Elizabeth's reign from 'an abundance of religion', others, like John Friar of Godmanchester, were happy to pay fines for their recusancy, while others became notorious for their Catholicism.[10] Balthasar Guercy, an Italian surgeon, had been imprisoned in 1543 for his pro-papal views, and spent the years 1551–4 in exile. Specifically excluded from the act of pardon because of his part in machinations against Archbishop Cranmer, he returned under Mary, became a Cambridge MD, and was elected to the college in December 1556, three weeks before his death.[11] Under Elizabeth Thomas Vavasour, who had taken his medical degree at Venice, was pursued throughout the north of England for his vigorous encouragement of his fellow Catholics.[12]

Closer to home, there were other friends who were at least suspected of adherence to Catholicism. The professor of rhetoric in Cambridge, Bartholomew Clerk (1537–1590), to whose Latin translation of Castiglione's *The Courtier* Caius contributed a preface in 1572, was accused of 'unsoundness in religion' in 1569, a charge from which he was cleared through the intervention of the Earl of Essex.[13] But friendship and collegiality do not of themselves indicate that Caius agreed with all that his friends and colleagues believed. Indeed, his reluctance to join Clement and others in exile brought down accusations from those abroad that he was a time-server, an opportunist who preferred to put his offices and reputation before adherence to the true faith.[14]

Philip Grierson argued from the evidence of the inventory of Caius' library that he was not a man of strong theological views, an interpretation refined by another great Caian historian, Christopher Brooke, who considered it improbable that he had 'thought deeply on theological topics'. But we cannot be sure that what was burned in 1572 did not contain some theological material. True, the inventory records no copies of such as Augustine, Aquinas or Nicholas of Lyra, but there are also other unexpected gaps, not least in medieval history, an area where Caius certainly carried out his own researches. His writings show no great interest in contemporary theological debates, but that is hardly surprising since for much of his life he was occupied almost entirely with college affairs, his medical practice and his writings on Galen and on the history of the institutions he served.

But there is a consistency in his religious outlook over most of his life that fits well with own description of his conservative mind-set as expounded in a typically rhetorical preface to his treatise on pronunciation. Over seven pages of vigorous Latin he defends his support for the old ways, whether in dress, university procedures or the pronunciation of Greek and Latin. All innovation, however good, may bring disaster in its wake, and nothing is worse than casting the old aside simply for the novelty of change. He reserves his praise for those who are not swept hither and thither on the tide of fashion, as in those universities where the flightiness of youth has led to frequent and confusing change, and the abandonment of tradition. A mighty array of classical authorities is assembled to substantiate his conviction that custom and habit are far less dangerous than innovation, which inevitably brings with it unexpected consequences. Although this diatribe could well be interpreted as an attack on religious developments, Caius is careful to specify that it refers only to non-religious matters, *in rebus civilibus dico*, which shows at least some awareness of the hazards of involvement in religious debate.[15]

Nonetheless, if we are to take seriously his professions of a conservative outlook on most things, it is his early theological writings that may give a clue to his beliefs, since they were written as a personal exercise and handed over to friends who had requested them. They all date from the 1530s, a period in Cambridge that Caius looked back to as a golden age in university life when contrasted with the turbulence he found when he returned in 1557. Many of the things with which he had been familiar had been swept away, and he found himself a stranger in a society that had abandoned deference and enthusiasm for scholarship in favour of outlandish fashions and games.[16] Much of this is wonderful rhetoric, yet it also reflects his own career as an undergraduate, a boy from Norwich who had risen swiftly through his own endeavours to become a fellow of his own college and the friend of leading prelates and courtiers.

His translations are typical of theological debate of the 1520s and early 1530s in their emphasis on the individual reaction to scripture, and its expression in personal prayer. It is very close to the ideas espoused by the great Christian humanist, Erasmus, whose residence in Cambridge between 1510 and 1515 would have been remembered by many of those with whom Caius was in contact. Indeed, two of Caius' translations were of works written by Erasmus, the *Paraphrase of Jude* and *The True Theology*. The former deals at length with the question of grace, warning against false prophets and those who have hypocritically 'crept like wolves into the sheepfold of the Lord'. The true Christian, strengthened by love of the gospel, will bring others to Christ by his own example and simple faith. This stress on personal piety gained by reading the New Testament was one of the main features of the second work of Erasmus, his *True Theology*, a *Method* of understanding the scriptures.[17] It was this aspect that attracted Caius to make a paraphrase rather than a complete English version, leaving out many of the subtleties that he thought were suitable only for 'great and learned divines' rather than for his patron, the Norwich Alderman, Augustine Stiward. In his much later *Autobibiography*, he adds the comment that he did this because Stiward did not know the appropriate boundaries of reading and studying the Scriptures or how to explore them 'safely'.[18] This adverb and the following sentence explaining that 'there was at that time a new form of religion beginning to spread widely in England,' certainly reflect Caius' views in 1570, and were shared by such as Archbishop Parker who were wary of the uncontrolled freedom of individuals to interpret scripture in their own way and of some of the radical interpretations being advanced, but they need not have been uppermost in Caius' mind when he produced his translation.[19]

A third translation, of Chrysostom's short tract on praying to God, was made from Erasmus' Latin version, which Caius turned into English to encourage friend at court 'who was not much given to prayer'.[20] Caius' Latin version from the Greek of 'a little boke of Nicephorus, declarynge how a man maye in praying confess hym selyfe', written for a young graduate called John Groome, also falls firmly within the Erasmian tradition, in that it uses a Byzantine patristic text to emphasise the importance of private prayers of confession, as opposed to the more formal auricular confession. Caius gives two different dates for its composition. In his treatise on the English Sweat he records that he began his translation activities when he was twenty, and places this version after his editing of the compositions of his late friend William Framingham, who died in September 1537. It is then followed by his *History of Norwich*. If this date is correct, the recipient would be John Groome, who graduated in 1536–37 and was briefly a fellow of St John's. However, in his much later *Autobibliography*, above, p. 54, he says that it was written in his twenty second year and was the first of his compositions, i.e. in 1530–31. If so, it would have been given to another John Groome, who graduated in 1529. Neither date is entirely satisfactory, but to adopt the later one would also involve placing the beginning of Caius' history of Norwich in the years shortly before his visit to Italy, which seems unlikely.

In either case, this was an unusual text to choose. It was a short text ascribed to an unfamiliar Byzantine theologian, Nicephorus Callistus Xanthopoulus, fl. 1320, and read by Caius in the original Greek.[21] As far as I am aware, there had been no printed edition of the Greek (or, for that matter, of any Latin version), and since Caius had yet to visit Italy, he must have found it in Cambridge or possibly in London. Since there is no evidence that any of the eight surviving manuscripts of this text had any connection with Britain, one must conclude that his manuscript is now lost. There is, however, a possible source, albeit tenuous. John Clement, whom Caius later knew very well and who was in many ways his model, not only owned a Greek manuscript of Chrysostom, *On Prayer*, but also translated some of the homilies of Callistus, presumably from a manuscript in his own extensive library.[22] This library, one of the largest of its day, was taken to the Continent during Clement's second period of exile and then subsequently dispersed in the Spanish sack of Malines in 1572. Although a handful of books and manuscripts from it have survived, the Callistus is not among them.

Caius' theological standpoint in the 1530s was one that would have been widely shared; an emphasis on personal piety, coupled with a sense of a Christian tradition that included the Greek as well as the Latin fathers, and saw nothing incongruous in embracing the ethical ideals of Ancient Greece and Rome. An emphasis on *virtus* instanced in his lament for the Swiss scholar Conrad Gessner as well as on his own tomb and that of Linacre in St Paul's did not indicate a retreat from Christianity, and only the most austere of theologians would have rejected a link between faith and good works.[23] A belief in the need for reform in the church, outlined by Erasmus and favoured by such as Cardinal Pole, was widespread in the 1530s, and Caius' work as a translator was neither very conservative nor revolutionary.

Certainly, in 1535, he saw no difficulty in subscribing to the Royal Supremacy along with most other members of Gonville Hall. Many of the senior fellows were sympathetic to Protestant doctrine, and several had strong links with the circle around Anne Boleyn, including the master, John Skippe, later bishop of Hereford. Caius himself regarded as one of his main patrons Sir William Butts, a royal physician widely viewed as a strong supporter of Protestant theologians at court. Many of those mentioned by Caius in this period can also be characterised as firm Protestants, like his great friend from Norwich, Matthew Parker, even if they might appear moderate by comparison with others in the 1560s. But there were equally others who held less advanced views or saw little reason to enter into controversies at all. Another main supporter, Sir Thomas Wendy, also a royal physician, remained more aloof from religious disputations. Caius flourished in such a community, and one can easily see why he should have looked back with such nostalgia to his first period in Cambridge.[24]

He was also fortunate that his time in Padua and his subsequent tour of Italian libraries came just before papal pressure began to make it increasingly dangerous for Protestants to travel around Italy. He mentions attending services of the Greek community in Venice and he may well have met Cardinal Pole, though there is no evidence for this. But as his *Autobibliography* makes clear, his links are with fellow scholars from both sides of the growing theological divide. He received help from numerous Italians, and claims friendship with internationally famous Protestants such as Melanchthon, Joachim Camerarius and Sebastian Münster, although, in Melanchthon's case, this may only have been an epistolary friendship or one conducted through intermediaries.

Annotations by Caius in his books reveal a little more about his private thoughts in the years after his return. In a note added to his 1544 edition of Galen's *Anatomical procedures* CULAdv, 1544: 2, he describes Henry VIII as 'defender of the faith in Christendom and supreme head of the church in Britain and Ireland'.[25] In a second note in his copy of the 1538 Basle edition of Galen, Etonadv I,α.2r, he pointedly declares that *aetas haec nostra tamen unicum habet principem henricum octavum doctum;* 'our age has only one learned prince, Henry VIII'. This note is difficult to date, but the hand is certainly later than that he used in Italy in the early 1540s, and is more akin to that in notes from the 1550s. But whether it was written before 1547 or, in a more critical vein, under Edward VI, this shows his high regard for Henry, and in the Cambridge annotation, his acceptance of the king's role as Defender of the Faith.[26] A further note in the Eton Galen, EtonAdv I,51, in a late hand probably of the 1550s, glosses Galen's reference to 'those who were sacking temples', with 'similarly in our time in Britain' (*tales nro tempore in Brit.*), which can hardly refer to events under Henry. His later comment on the need for those reading the scriptures to know the boundaries of interpretation, above, p. 54, can also be taken as a criticism of evangelicals.

These notes only confirm what could easily have been surmised, that John Caius was on the conservative end of the spectrum of belief in the 1540s, but also that he was happy with the idea of a Royal Supremacy over an ordered church. His regard for Henry would only have been strengthened by the actions he took against the evangelicals in the last years of his reign. But at the same time, there is nothing here that would not have been accepted by the great majority of Christians in England nor would his support for a non-papal Catholicism have marked him out, as yet, as one strongly opposed to every change. There is little doubt also that he approved of the accession of Mary and the return of Cardinal Pole, and he benefited from their support in re-founding his college and in his attempts to impose the writ of the London College of Physicians on its competitors.[27] But he was not so zealous a Catholic as to be immediately suspect when Elizabeth came to the throne and instituted a visitation of her universities. Besides, although she reversed many of her sister's measures, her reluctance to agree to all that the returned evangelicals had desired, as well as her support for his friend Archbishop Parker, would have reassured Caius in the maintenance of his conservative stance.[28] He was not alone in this, even in Cambridge, and recent research has only emphasised how slowly evangelical doctrines and practices penetrated the wider Christian community in England.[29]

Ceri Law in her study of religious change in Cambridge in this period also draws attention to Caius' role in wider university affairs.[30] Only recently appointed Master of his college with the enthusiastic support of both college and university, he knew many of the Commissioners appointed by Elizabeth to review the university in summer, 1559. As well as Matthew Parker and Thomas Wendy, he mentions Sir Anthony Cooke in his *Autobibliography*, and both William Bill and Walter Haddon had friends in common with him, and would have been well placed to judge whether he was among the 'lazy, idle and culpable persons, and those who obstinately and peremptorily refuse to subscribe to the religion which we have now received in its amended form.' Nor was Caius one of the two Masters of colleges that Robert Beaumont advised Cecil in 1561 should be removed to allow pure religion to take better root. Three years later, he played a leading role in the disputations when the queen visited the university – not entirely to the queen's satisfaction, for his thin, hig,h squeaky voice made him almost inaudible and the queen had to leave her chair to come closer to him.[31] His interest in medieval documents and the history of the university also made him a useful participant in the revision of the university statutes in 1570.[32] At the very least, all this suggests that either the pressure on Cambridge to reform in the early 1560s was less than in Oxford or that Caius' religious views, allied to his willingness to conform, did not, as yet, present serious difficulties. Besides, for perhaps a decade more at least, many of Elizabeth's subjects, not least in Cambridge, adhered to the beliefs and ceremonies of the old religion. They would have sympathised with his desire to be buried close to a site in the chapel where once stood a tabernacle housing an image of our Lady.[33]

Law has suggested that local tensions within both the university and the close-knit communities of individual colleges contributed a good deal to accusations of popery. Caius' relations with his colleagues and undergraduates were never easy, at least in his early years, and resulted in several letters of complaint to the authorities. His desire that 'his' fellows and scholars should always abide by his wishes and his statutes easily slipped into somewhat petulant and overbearing action that led to expulsions and in at least one case to a period of imprisonment.[34] In 1572 several members of the college joined in the complaints and in the ransacking of his rooms, although he himself attributed everything to the hostility of a single student. Similar internal disputes in King's College had twice led to formal complaints to the chancellor about the behaviour and papist beliefs of the provost, Philip Baker, which resulted in his flight abroad in 1569.

Baker's case contrasts with that of Bartholomew Clerk already mentioned and with that of Caius. Both the others enjoyed the support of leading figures in the religious politics of the time, Clerk from the earl of Essex, Caius from both Cecil and Archbishop Parker. The latter's friendship with Caius went back to Norwich days, and they shared many interests, not least in history. Caius made Parker his literary executor, and he relied on members of Parker's circle in some at least of his historical works on the university of Cambridge.[35] His account of a dinner with Parker and Bishop Guest of Rochester shows that he still enjoyed their company in the years immediately before the catastrophe. At times both Parker and Cecil found his behaviour annoying – but that of some of his detractors even more so. Others were less sympathetic to the old man. Bishop Parkhurst, in a letter dated 4 March, 1568, reported to a friend in Zurich that the queen instructed some of her councillors to eject papists from the court 'to the great joy of the godly', and in the next sentence, that she had told Parker to do the same with his household.[36] A slightly later hand adds in the margin the name of John Caius, although his inclusion, like the story of his dismissal as a royal physician, seems to be little more than rumour. Parker's final letters to the dying Caius reveal their closeness, as well as the compassion with which the archbishop responded to his old friend. More ambiguous is Cecil's brief reference to Caius, 'whose Sowle god pardon', in his letter of January 1574 to the fellows of Caius instructing them to elect a successor. This somewhat old-fashioned phrase may have been chosen out of respect for his old friend and his colleagues rather than used ironically.[37]

Caius' liking for an older form of religion was, it is now clear, shared by many in Cambridge and beyond. His *Autobibliography* of 1570 presents a confident picture of a scholar, 'senior, but not senile', with friends and acquaintances around Europe, from Catholic exiles to leading Protestants. When he finished it in early 1570, he still had plans for the future. There were editions of Galen to complete, as well as his history of Norwich. His rebuilding of his college was almost finished, and some of the turbulence of earlier years had abated. In this time of felicity, he may not have appreciated how quickly the situation might change. Some of the pressure came from outside Cambridge. The pope's excommunication of Queen Elizabeth in 1570 gave a further opportunity for those who wished to identify papist belief and practices with political disloyalty, and the growing strength of evangelicals at court and on the episcopal bench meant less tolerance for those who thought differently within the Anglican church. Ceri Law has also emphasised the role played by disputes within individual Cambridge Colleges, where personal dislikes, as well as magisterial attempts to impose greater conformity, provided ample opportunity for outsiders to be involved in a wider conflict.

Gonville and Caius College, and Thomas Legge, Caius' friend and successor as Master, long retained a reputation for popish views, but, although further protests led to an investigation ordered by the chancellor in 1580, there was no repetition of the catastrophe of 1572.[38] Indeed, several of those involved in the raid of 1572 played leading parts in the funeral ceremonies of 1573, going out to the Trumpington ford to accompany the body back, a sign of respect on the part of the university authorities. Likewise, the fellows of Caius were quick to respond to Caius' requests from London for books to be sent to him in early 1573.[39] That the situation remained fluid is indicated by the praise lavished on Caius only four years later by the translator of his *De canibus*, Abraham Fleming. The Latin preface, dedicated to the great Cambridge survivor Andrew Perne, talks of his extremely close friendship with Caius, the 'shining light, jewel and glory of the university of Cambridge'.[40] The address to the reader is even more effusive in its eulogy of Caius, 'a profound clarke and a ravennous deuourer of learning', whose lament for Gessner is taken as a sign of his own moral stature. Distance, and the death of Caius, can account for the change of tone from the vituperations of 1572, although Fleming hints that others might see things differently.[41]

That Caius was a self-confessed conservative is undeniable. He could accept the royal headship of the church in England, while at the same time seeking to retain as much as possible of the ornaments and practices of the church catholic. He was not alone in this, as recent scholarship has abundantly emphasised, but his position in Cambridge laid him open to challenges that were more specifically religious than those he had faced in London. In his own college he could use his authority to stifle dissent, not always to universal satisfaction, and as others found, local divisions had a way of becoming more significant. But up into the 1570s he could see himself as secure. A friend of many distinguished figures across the religious spectrum, a scholar of international repute and protected on more than one occasion by the archbishop of Canterbury and the chancellor of the university, he could remain optimistic and look forward to several more years of productive activity.[42] The ransacking of his rooms in December 1572 will thus have come as a great shock, and contributed, so his friends believed, to his ill health and to his death only a few months later. His last writings, and the records of his final months, show how much he continued to believe in an Erasmian unity of Christian and humanist values that stretched back to the early church and that cut across confessional boundaries. The roots of his misfortune may well have lain in his failure to recognise the generational differences and the change of tone in the wider community that turned scholarly disagreements into religious and ultimately political ones.[43] It was a catastrophe that those who had supported him were no longer able to prevent.[44]

Notes

1 Venn (1912: 26–7); Brooke (1985: 76), spelling slightly modernised. The letter of complaint dated by Venn (1912: 26) to 1565 is re-dated by Grierson (1978: 524, n. 10) to 1572/3.

2 Above, p. 54.

3 Nutton (2017b). The extent to which it was revised after 1570, when it is mentioned in his *Autobibliography*, above, p. 124, is unclear. At Caius 1574d: 4 = 4 R., Caius says that it was finished in 1573. The published version includes the names of Thomas Byng, Master of Clare in 1571, Robert Norgate, Master of Corpus Christi in 1573, and Thomas Legge, installed as Master of Caius only a few days before Caius' death.

4 Ibid., p. 15 = 12 R.

5 Ibid., p. 65 = 52 R. Christopher Brooke reminded me that the names and formal titles of both monarchs open the beautiful charter authorising the refoundation of Gonville Hall, see Caius, *Annals of Gonville and Caius College*, pp. 43, 61.

6 Ibid., p. 131 = 106 R., Thomas Cromwell is described as becoming Chancellor 'after the death of the Bishop of Rochester', i.e. John Fisher.

7 Ibid., p. 59 = 47 R. North's deathbed (re-)conversion to Catholicism was well known. Caius himself was a great admirer of Chrysostom's theology, but Lupset's friendship with Cardinal Pole will also have been remembered.

8 Ibid., p. 124 = 100 R. Note his association of Edward VI with the losses of his Cambridge College through currency devaluation in 1551. Similar losses in 1560 and 1561 are not attributed to Elizabeth (Caius 1904: 81–2).

9 Caius' friend Conrad Gessner assumed that George Bullock, Master of St John's and an exile on the Continent from 1559, would easily be able to deliver a message to Caius; in fact, Bullock was on his way to Italy.

10 The phrase is applied by George Lewkenor (Woolfson 1998: 251) to his friend, Edward, 3rd Lord Windsor, d. 1575, on the epitaph he composed for him in the church of SS. Giovanni e Paolo in Venice. For Friar, see Woolfson (1998: 238).

11 Munk (1878: 57); Bennell (2004b).

12 Munk (1878: 56–7); Palmer (1983: 137); Rex (1990–91, 2004b).

13 Caius (1585: 11–12); British Library, Sloane MS 3562, 15r-v, 21r-v, details the case against Clerk.

14 Pitseus (1619: 755–6), depending in part on information from the Clement family, describes him as 'unsound in faith, an opportunist, constantly changing his mind one way or the other'. Duffy (2009: 201) has no hesitation in calling him a notorious cryptopapist, but this is to underestimate his attachment to his roots.

15 Caius (1574: 2–9 = 4–8 R.)

16 Caius (1574: 3 = 3 R.)

17 Boyle (1977).

18 For the recipient, Alderman Augustine Stiward of Norwich, see above, p. 54. Erasmus' *Ratio verae theologiae*, 'the true and redye way to reade the scripture', was first published at Louvain in 1518 by T. Martens, but Caius may well have used the enlarged edition, Basle: Froben, 1520. It was a substantial work, and one can see why Caius should have wished to summarize it. In the *English Sweat* (1552: 4 = 5 R.), Caius says that he left out 'many subtile things made rather for great & learned diuines, thē for others.' No copy of any of the theological works here listed appears in the inventory of his library.

19 This is a sideswipe at the Lutheran ideas that had flourished in Cambridge in the 1530s, and were later to lead to the evangelical puritanism that he disliked.

20 John Chrysostom, *Homily* 6, on prayer. For the importance of prayer in Erasmus' theology, see Pabel (1997).

21 Nicephorus Callistus, fl. 1320, was a Byzantine cleric and historian, remembered today largely for his *Ecclesiastical History*, but the author also of religious works (Jugie 1931, but with no mention of this tract). This small text survives today in only eight manuscripts (http://pinakes.irht.cnrs.fr/notices/oeuvre/11583: accessed 11/8/2017), none of which can Caius have known.

22 Wenkebach (1925: 28, 68); Reed (1925–26: 337), emending '*riantes*' to '*orantes*'.

23 For Linacre's tomb, see Venn (1912: 11). One should not categorise Caius' interest in angels, familiar spirits, visions, mirrors and magic, British Library, Add. 36, 674, ff. 20r–45v, found among his 'secret writings' as incompatible with a Christian belief. It is typical of that of a learned man of the period.

24 The list of names who read Caius' edition of Framingham's poems, above, p. 7, reveals something of the East Anglian/Norfolk group of Henrician supporters to which he was connected.

25 'fidei defenso[ri]/ atque in terris/ secundum chri[stum] ecclesiae Brit[an]/nicae et Hib[er]/nicae suprem[o] capiti'. He also in the headings of the preface thought of calling Henry 'nobilissimus', but then deleted the word.

26 This point is not affected by Bernard's argument (2005) that Henry was intent on carrying out more fully an evangelical reformation: actions taken against Lutheran sympathisers and the exile of several prominent Cambridge figures would only have encouraged those who believed that Henry had changed his mind.

27 Above, p. 21.

28 Marshall (2017: 48–54) provides a clear summary of the ambiguities of the Elizabethan settlement. Ceri Law suggests to me that the shortness of the reigns of both Edward and Mary only added to the uncertainty about what might happen if Elizabeth were to die similarly inopportunely, and that is was not foolish to refrain from disposing of vestments and the like immediately. Elizabeth herself preferred a more Catholic ritual in her private chapel, to the annoyance of many of her bishops. Cf. also McGrath (1967: 47–99, labelling the period 1558–1570 as 'the years of uncertainty'); Walsham (2014: 53–102).

29 Porter (1958: 209), suggesting that in 1570 half the university might have been sympathetic to Caius' views; Shuger (2009: 606–7) rightly seeing Caius as a representative figure of Anglican belief; Law (2018 ,ch. 6). Cf. Walsham (1999: 20): 'Until the 1570s at least, the Church of England largely proved a tolerable substitute for, if an inferior version of, its medieval predecessor.'

30 For the wider background of university affairs, see Morgan (2004: 63–96).

31 His participation would have been ill advised if, as is often asserted, he had been a Royal physician dismissed for his religious views. No evidence has so far been produced that he ever held such a position – he is not mentioned in any disbursements in the Royal Household – and his comment in the *Annals of the College of*

Physicians: 59 R., that Robert Huyck stepped down as president in 1564 because of his commitments as a royal physician, implies that he too would not have wished to combine both posts.

32 Venn (1912: 53).

33 Venn (1912: 73).

34 Venn (1912: 23–6, 54).

35 Grafton (2017).

36 Cambridge University Library, Ms. Ee.ii.34, f. 7. Houlbrooke's translation (1974: 62) leaves it unclear as to which sentence the anonymous annotator was referring, but the Latin is unambiguous.

37 Law (2018).

38 Contrast Brooke (1985: 89–93), emphasising that Legge became vice-chancellor in 1587–8, with Law (2018: ch. 6), arguing for the significance of the intervention of Sir Christopher Hatton in changing Cecil's mind in 1580.

39 Venn (1912: 40), a point I owe to Michael Prichard.

40 Caius (1576: pf = np. R.): '*Cantabrigiensis academiae lumen, gemma, et gloria.*'.

41 Ibid.: 49–50 = np. R., preface to the reader, although the statement that 'the mouth of th'adversary must needes confesse & giue sentence that commendation ought to bee his rewarde, and praise his deserued pension' could also be taken as a mere literary trope.

42 His friend Richard Willison in a letter of April, 1572 (Venn: 1912, 43) writes of 'calumpniators', who, he suggests, were envious of his 'vertuous enterprises', but this may be a hint of things to come.

43 John Strype (1821: 155) saw no difficulty in attributing Caius' views on Greek pronunciation to his popery.

44 Nonetheless, it did not lead to any formal charges against him, to his deposition as master or as with Philip Baker, to exile, but only to a withdrawal to London.

Bibliography

Abbreviations

BNF Bibliothèque nationale de France.

CMG *Corpus medicorum Graecorum* (1914–). Leipzig and Berlin: Teubner, Akademie Verlag, W. De Gruyter.

CULAdv *Galeni medici libri aliquot graeci*. Basle: H. Froben and N. Episcopius, 1544, now Cambridge University Library, Adv.d.3.1 (formerly Nn.3.19).

DBI *Dizionario biografici degli Italiani* (1960–). Rome: Treccani.

EtonAdv *Galeni Pergameni. . . . Opera omnia*. Basle: H. Froben, 1538, now Eton College Library, Fc.2.6–8.

K. Kühn KG (1821–1832) *Claudii Galeni opera omnia*. Leipzig: K. Knobloch.

L. Littré E (1839–61) *Oeuvres complètes d'Hippocrate*. Paris: J.B. Baillière.

ODNB *Oxford Dictionary of National Biography* (2004–). Oxford: Oxford University Press, 2004–; UPDATEonline edn, consulted September 2017.

R. Roberts ES (ed.) (1912) *The Works of John Caius, M.D., Second Founder of Gonville and Caius College and Master of the College 1559–1573*. Cambridge: Cambridge University Press.

Bibliography

The published works of John Caius

(An asterisk indicates that the work is reprinted in Roberts 1912.)

1544a *De medendi methodo libri duo, ex Cl. Galeni Pergameni & Jo. Baptistae Montani Veronensis, principum medicorum sententia*. Basle: H. Froben and N. Episcopius.

1544b *Galeni medici libri aliquot graeci*. Basle: H. Froben and N. Episcopius.

1549 *Galeni De sanitate tuenda*. Basle: H. Froben.

1552 *A Boke or Counseill against the Disease commonly called the Sweate or Sweatyng Sicknesse*. London: R. Grafton.*

1556 *Opera aliquot et versiones, partim jam nata, partim recognita atque aucta*. Louvain: A.M. Bergagne.

[Contains a slightly revised version of 1544a,* *De ephemera Britannica*,* and his translations of Galen's *De libris suis, De ordine librorum suorum, De ratione victus secundum Hippocratem in morbis acutis*, and *De placitis Hippocratis et Platonis*, Book I.]

1557 *Galeni Pergameni Libri. De septimestri partu. Brevis designatio dogmatum Hippocratis. De ptisana. De ossibus. Integri et emendati*. Basle: J. Oporinus.

1568 *De antiquitate Cantebrigiensis academiæ libri duo, Londinensi authore* [J. Caius]. *Adiunximus assertionem antiquitatis Oxoniensis academiæ, ab Oxoniensi quodam* [T. Caius] *conscriptam.* London: H. Bynneman.

1570a,b,c *De canibus Britannicis, liber unus.* *De rariorum animalium et stirpium historia, liber unus.* *De libris propriis, liber unus.* London: W. Seres.

1574a,b,c,d *De antiquitate Cantebrigiensis academiæ libri duo, Londinensi authore* [J. Caius].* *Adiunximus assertionem antiquitatis Oxoniensis academiæ, ab Oxoniensi quodam* [T. Caius] *conscriptam. Historia Cantebrigiensis academiae ab urbe condita.* *De pronunciatione Graecae & Latinae linguae cum scriptione nova libellus.* London: J. Day* [Printed together with separate pagination.]

1576 *Of Englishe Dogges, the diuersities, the names, the natures and the properties. A short treatise written in latine by Johannes Caius . . . and newly drawne into Englishe by Abraham Fleming. B.L.* London: Rychard Johnes.*

1577 *Balthasaris Castilionis Comitis De curiali siue aulico libri quatuor, ex Italico sermone in Latinum conuersi. Bartholomæo Clerke Anglo Cantabrigiensi interprete.* London: H. Bynneman.

1585 *Balthasaris Castilionis Comitis De curiali siue aulico libri quatuor, ex Italico sermone in Latinum conuersi. Bartholomæo Clerke Anglo Cantabrigiensi interprete.* London: T. Dauson.

1729 *De canibus Britannicis, liber unus.* *De rariorum animalium et stirpium historia, liber unus.* *De libris propriis, liber unus.* London: Charles Davis.

1904 *The Annals of Gonville and Caius College Cambridge, edited by John Venn. Publications of the Cambridge Antiquarian Society, 40.* Cambridge: Cambridge Antiquarian Society.

1912 *The First Book of the Annals of the Royal College of Physicians, London . . . comprising the Years 1518–1572.*

Roberts ES (ed) (1912) *The Works of John Caius*, M.D., *Second Founder of Gonville and Caius College and Master of the College 1559–1573.* Cambridge, Cambridge University Press.

Annotations

1538 *Galeni Pergameni. . . . Opera omnia.* Basle: H. Froben, now Eton College Library, Fc.2.6–8.

1544 *Galeni medici libri aliquot graeci.* Basle: H. Froben and N. Episcopius, now Cambridge University Library, Adv.d.3.1 (formerly Nn.3.19).

Secondary works

Adolph A (2015) *Brutus of Troy and the Quest for the Ancestry of the British.* Barnsley: Pen and Sword Family History.

Agasse JM and Pennuto C (eds) (2016) *Girolamo Mercuriale, Johann Crato von Kraffiheim. Une correspondance entre deuz médecins humanistes.* Geneva: Droz.

Agnelli G (1932) Biblioteche della Provincia di Ferrara. In Fava D (ed) *Emilia e Romagna.* Milan: U. Hoepli: 39–80.

Agrimi J and Crisciani C (1988) Edocere medicos. In *Medicina scolastica nei secoli XIII–XV.* Naples: Guerini e Associati.

——— (1994) *Les Consilia médicaux. Typologie des sources du Moyen Âge occidental.* Turnhout: Brepols.

Alce V and D'Amato A (1961) *La biblioteca di San Domenico in Bologna.* Florence: L. S.Olschki.

Alexandrinus J (1548) *Galeni enantiomaton aliquot liber*. Venice: Giunta.

Allen PS (ed) (1906–1958) *Opus epistolarum Des. Erasmi Roterodami*. Oxford: Clarendon Press.

André J (1991) *Le vocabulaire de l'anatomie*. Paris: Les Belles Lettres.

Andretta E (2011) *Roma medica. Anatomie d'un système médical au XVIᵉsiécle*. Paris: École française de Rome.

Anon. (1959) *An Inventory of the Historical Monuments in the City of Cambridge*. London: Royal Commission on Historical Monuments.

Aquilecchia G (1999) L'esperienze anglo-scozzese di Cardano e l'inquisizione. In Baldi M and Canziani G (eds) *Girolamo Cardano, Le opere, le fonti, la vita*. Milan: FrancoAngeli: 379–91.

Arbenz E (ed) (1891) *Die Vadianische Briefsammlung der Stadtbibliothek St. Gallen, II, Mitteilungen zur vaterländische Geschichte*, 25.2. St. Gallen: St Gallen Historischer Verein.

Archer IW (2004) Smith, Sir Thomas. In *ODNB* 51: 323–30.

Armitage CM (2009) Dr Caius: Cambridge Scholar, Shakespearean Buffoon. In *Notes and Queries* 56.1: 46–8.

Avesani R (1960) Amaseo, Pompilio. In *DBI* 2: 658–66.

——— (1969) Bonamico, Lazzaro. In *DBI* 11: 533–40.

Baltussen HN (ed) (2013) *Greek and Roman Consolations: Eight Studies of a Tradition and Its Afterlife*. Swansea: The Classical Press of Wales.

Barcia Goyanes JJ (1982) *Onomatologia anatomica nova. Historia del lenguaje anatómico, Tomo V. Ligamentum talonaviculare – myometrium*. Valencia: Universidad de Valencia, Secretariado de Publicationes.

Baron F (ed) (1978) *Joachim Camerarius (1500–1574). Essays on the History of Humanism During the Reformation*. Munich: Funk.

Bartholin T (1667a) *Epistolarum medicinalium centuria III. Variis observationibus curiosis et utilibus referta*. Copenhagen: M. Godicchenius for P. Haubold.

——— (1667b) *Epistolarum medicinalium centuria IV. Variis observationibus curiosis et utilibus referta*. Copenhagen: M. Godicchenius for P. Haubold.

——— (1670) *De Bibliothecae incendio dissertatio ad filios*. Copenhagen: M. Godicchenius.

Bateman JJ (trans) (1993) *Erasmus, Paraphrase on the Epistle of Jude: Collected Works of Erasmus*, vol. 44. Toronto, Buffalo and London: University of Toronto Press: 123–30.

Beer BL (2004) Hatcher, Thomas (*d*. 1583). In *ODNB* 25: 802–3.

Beilin EV (ed) (2009) *Early Tudor Women Writers*. Farnham and Burlington, VT: Ashgate.

Bennell J (2004a) Browne, Lancelot. In *ODNB* 8: 180–1.

——— (2004b) Guercy, Balthasar. In *ODNB* 24: 167.

Berengario da Carpi J (1521) *Commentaria. . . . Super Anatomia Mundini*. Bologna: H.de Benedictis.

——— (1522) *Isagoge breves . . . in anatomiam humani corporis*. Bologna: H.de Benedictis.

Berlier S (2011) John Caius et le 'De usu partium'. Contribution à l'histoire du texte de Galien. In *Revue d'histoire des textes* 6: 1–14.

Bernard GW (2005) *The King's Reformation. Henry VIII and the Remaking of the English Church*. New Haven and London: Yale University Press.

Beroaldo F (1487) *Commentarii in Propertium*. Bologna: B. Hectoris and P. De Benedictis.

Blair A (2017) The Dedication Strategies of Conrad Gessner. In Manning G and Klestinec C (eds) *Professors, Physicians and Practices in the History of Medicine:*

Essays in Honor of Nancy Siraisi. Archimedes 50. n.p.: Springer International: 169–209.

Blume F (1827) *Iter Italicum. Zweiter Band. Archive, Bibliotheken und Inschriften in Parma, Modena, Massa, Lucca, Toscana, dem Kirchenstaat und S. Marino.* Halle: E. Anton.

Boissard J J (1588) *Emblematum liber.* Metz: J. Aubry.

Bonazza M (2003) Percorsi storici di una biblioteca nata nel secolo dell' Encyclopedie. In Toselli AF (ed) *La Biblioteca pubblica di Ferrara: 250 anni di libri e lettori.* Ferrara: Centro stampa Comune di Ferrara: 1753–2003.

Bonorand C (1980) *Joachim Vadian und der Humanismus im Bereich des Erzbistums Salzburg.* St. Gallen: Fehr'sche Buchhandlung.

Borsetti F (1735) *Historia almi Ferrariae gymnasii.* Ferrara: Bernardino Pomatelli.

Bosman-Jelgersma HA (ed) (1996a) *Pieter Van Foreest. De Hollandse Hippocrates.* Krommenie: Drukkerij Knijnenberg.

———— (ed) (1996b) *Petrus Forestus medicus.* Duivendrecht: Drukkerij Stolwijk.

Boudon-Millot V (1999) John Caius (1510–1573) traducteur de Galien: le cas du De libris propriis et du De ordine librorum suorum. In Garzya A and Jouanna J (eds) *I testi medici greci.Tradizione e ecdotica, Atti del III Convegno Internazionale (Napoli, 15–18 ottobre 1997).* Naples: M. d'Auria Editore: 17–27.

———— (2007) *Galien. Tome I. Introduction générale. Sur l'ordre de ses propres livres. Sur ses propres livres. Que l'excellent médecin est aussi philosophe.* Paris: Les Belles Lettres.

———— and Cobolet G (eds) (2004) *Lire les médecins grecs à la Renaissance: aux origines de l'édition médicale: actes du colloque international de Paris, 19–20 septembre 2003.* Paris: Bibliothèque interuniversitaire de médecine.

Bowden CMK (2004) Cecil, Mildred. In *ODNB* 10: 743–5.

———— (2009) The Library of Mildred Cecil, Lady Burghley. In Beilin EV (ed) *Early Tudor Women.* Farnham and Burlington, VT: Ashgate: 399–426.

Bowker M (2004a) Clement, Margaret. In *ODNB* 12: 22.

———— (2004b) Roper, Margaret. In *ODNB* 47: 718–19.

———— (2004c) Taylor, John. In *ODNB* 53: 929–30.

Boyle MO'R (1977) *Erasmus on Language and Method in Theology.* Toronto and Buffalo: University of Toronto Press.

Brinckhus G and Pachnicke C (eds) (2001) *Leonhart Fuchs 1501–1566. Mediziner und Botaniker.* Tübingen: Stadtmuseum.

Brooke CNL (1985) *A History of Gonville and Caius College.* Woodbridge: The Boydell Press.

Brown P (2013) Terence and Greek Comedy. In Augoustakis A and Traill A (eds) *A Companion to Terence.* Chichester: Wiley Blackwell: 17–32.

Bruun CW (1893) *Paa hundrede-aarsdagen efter at det store kongelige bibliothek. Heri Johan Rode, født i København 1587, død i Padua 1659.* Copenhagen: Thieles Bogtrykkeri.

Burmann P (ed) (1727) *Sylloges epistolarum a viris illustribus scriptarum tomus quintus.* Leiden: S. Luchtmans.

Bylebyl JJ (1991) Teaching *Methodus Medendi* in the Renaissance. In Kudlien F and Durling RJ (eds) *Galen's Method of Healing. Proceedings of the 1982 Galen Symposium. Studies in Ancient Medicine* 1. Leiden and New York: E. J. Brill: 157–89.

Cagliuso DM (2015) *Progressive Reactionary: The Life and Works of John Caius, MD.* B.Phil. Diss., University of Pittsburgh.

Calvi FM (1525) *Hippocratis octaginta volumina, quibus maxima ex parte annorum circiter duo millia Latina caruit lingua.* Rome: FM Calvi.

Cardano G (1663) *Opera omnia*. Lyons: Jean Antoine Huguetan and Marc Antoine Ravaud.

Cavill PR (2013) Heresy and Forfeiture in Marian England. In *The Historical Journal* 56: 879–907.

Cerroni M (2003) Guarini, Alessandro. In *DBI* 60: 333–4.

Cheke J (1555) *De pronuntiatione Graecae potissimum linguae disputationes cum Stephano Vintonensi Episcopo*. Basle: N. Episcopius.

Clark Sir G. (1964) *A History of the Royal College of Physicians*. Oxford: Clarendon Press, for the Royal College of Physicians.

Colombo R (1559) *De re anatomica*. Venice: N. Bevilacqua.

Corti M (1550) *In Mundini Anatomen Explicatio*. Pavia: F. Moscheno and G.B. Negro.

Craik EM (2006) *Two Hippocratic Treatises On Sight and On Anatomy*. Leiden and Boston: Brill.

——— (2009) *The Hippocratic Treatise On Glands*. Leiden and Boston: Brill.

——— (2015) *The 'Hippocratic' Corpus. Content and Context*. London and New York: Routledge.

Crankshaw DJ and Gillespie A (2004) Parker, Matthew (1504–1575). In *ODNB* 42: 707–28.

Crato J (1555) *Methodus θεραπευτικη, ex sententia Galeni et Joannis Baptistae Montani*. Basle: J. Oporinus.

——— (1563) *In Cl. Galeni diuinos libros Methodi therapeutices Perioche methodica*. Basle: P. Perna.

Crawford J (2010) Literary Circles and Communities. In Bick C and Summit J (eds) *The History of British Women's Writing, 1500–1610*. London: Macmillan: 34–59.

Creighton C (1891) *A History of Epidemics in Britain From AD 664 to the Extinction of Plague*. Cambridge: Cambridge University Press.

D'Amato A (1988) *I Domenicani e l'Università di Bologna*. Bologna: ESD.

Da Monte GB (1558) *Opuscula varia ac praeclara*. Basle: M. Isingrin for P. Perna.

Danzi M (2016) Gessner balnéologue. In Leu UB and Ruoss M (eds) *Facetten eines Universums. Conrad Gessner 1516–2016*. Zurich: Neue Züricher Zeitung: 119–28.

Davies J (2009) *Culture and Power: Tuscany and Its Universities 1537–1609*. Leiden and Boston: Brill.

Debus AG (1965) *The English Paracelsians*. London: Oldbourne.

De Ferrari A (1983) Corti, Matteo. In *DBI* 29: 795–7.

De Lacy P (ed) (1978–1984) *On the Doctrines of Plato and Hippocrates. Edition, Translation and Commentary. CMG* V 4,1,2. Berlin: Akademie Verlag.

Delisle C (2008) *Establishing the Facts: Conrad Gessner's Epistolae Morales Between the Particular and the General*. Ph.D. Diss., University of London.

Devreesse R (1965) *Le fonds grec de la Bibliothèque vaticane des origines à Paul V*. Vatican City: Biblioteca apostolica vaticana.

Dowling M (1997) The Gospel and the Court: Reformation Under Henry VIII. In Lake P and Dowling M (eds) *Protestantism in the National Church in Sixteenth-century England*. London: Croom Helm.

Ducceschi V (1929–1930) Un epistolario inedito di dotti padovani della prima metà del Sec. XVIII. In *Atti e Memorie della R. Accademia di Scienze, Letter e Arti in Padova, n.s.* 46: 317–23.

Duckworth WHL, Lyons MC and Towers B (trans) (1962) *Galen On Anatomical Procedures. The Later Books*. Cambridge: Cambridge University Press.

Duffy E (2009) *Fires of Faith. Catholic England Under Mary Tudor*. New Haven and London: Yale University Press.

Durling RJ (1961) A Chronological Census of Renaissance Editions and Translations of Galen. In *Journal of the Warburg and Courtauld Institutes* 24: 230–305.

Egmond F (2013) A Collection Within a Collection. Rediscovered Animal Drawings From the Collections of Conrad Gessner and Felix Platter. In *Journal of the History of Collections* 25.2: 149–70.

———— (2016) Animal Drawings From Gessner's *Historia Animalium* Rediscovered in Amsterdam. In Leu UB and Ruoss M (eds) *Facetten eines Universums: Conrad Gessner 1516–1565*. Zürich: Verlag Neue Züricher Zeitung: 155–62.

Eloy NFJ (1764) *Dizionario storico della medicina*. Naples: Benedetto Gessari.

Erasmus D (1528) *De recta latini graecique sermonis pronunciatione*. Basle: Froben.

Eriksson R (1959) *Andreas Vesalius' First Public Anatomy at Bologna 1540: An Eyewitness Report by Baldasar Heseler Medicinae Scolaris Together With His Notes on Matthaeus Curtius' Lectures on Anatomia Mundini*. Uppsala and Stockholm: Almqvist and Wiksell.

Evans RJW (1973) *Rudolf II and His World: A Study in Intellectual History 1576–1612*. Oxford: Clarendon Press.

Fallopius H (1561) *Observationes anatomicae*. Venice: M. A. Ulmus.

Fay I (2015) *Health and the City: Disease, Environment and Government in Norwich, 1200–1575*. Woodbridge: Boydell and Brewer.

Ferretto S (2012) *Maestri per il metodo di trattar le cose. Bassiano Lando, Giovan Battista da Monte e la scienza della medicina nel xvi secolo*. Padua: CLEUP.

Fierz M (1983) *Girolamo Cardano, 1501–1576*. Boston: Birkhäuser.

Findlen P (1994) *Possessing Nature. Museums, Collecting and Scientific Culture in Early Modern Italy*. Berkeley, Los Angeles and London: University of California Press.

Fisher E (2008) Planoudes' *De trinitate*, the Art of Translation, and the Beholder's Share. In Demacopoulos G and Papanikolaou A (eds) *Orthodox Readings of Augustine*. Crestwood, NY: St. Vladimir's Press: 41–61.

Fletcher JM (1977) Linacre's Lands and Lectureships. In Maddison F, Pelling M and Webster C (eds) *Essays on the Life and Work of Thomas Linacre c.1460–1524*. Oxford: Clarendon Press: 107–77.

Formentin M (1978) *I codici greci di medicina nelle Tre Venezie*. Padua: Liviana.

Forrester JM and Henry J (2005) *Jean Fernel's on the Hidden Causes of Things*. Leiden: Brill.

Fortuna S (2005) Galeno Latino, 1490–1533. *Medicina nei secoli* 17: 469–506.

———— (2012) The Latin Editions of Galen's *Opera omnia* (1490–1625) and Their Prefaces. In *Early Science and Medicine* 17: 391–412.

Foxe J (1563) *Actes & Monuments of These Perillous Dayes*. London: J. Day.

Fraenkel E (2007) *Plautine Elements in Plautus*. Oxford: Oxford University Press.

Franceschini A (1970) *Nuovi documenti relativi ai docenti dello Studio di Ferrara nel sec. XVI. Deputazione provinciale Ferrarese di Storia Patria, Monumenti VI*. Ferrara: SATE.

Freeman J (2004) Guest, Edmund (1514–1577). In *ODNB* 24: 170–1.

French RK (1979) *De Juvamentis Membrorum* and the Reception of Galenic Physiological Anatomy. In *Isis* 70: 96–109.

———— (1999) *Dissection and Vivisection in the European Renaissance*. Aldershot: Ashgate.

———— and Lloyd GER (1978) Greek Fragments of the Lost Books of Galen's *Anatomical Procedures*. In *Sudhoffs Archiv* 62: 235–49.

Fuchs L (1531) *Compendiaria ac succincta admodum in artem medendi. . . . introductio*. Hagenau: J. Secerius.

―――― (1541) *Methodus seu ratio compendiaria cognoscendi veram solidamque medicinam*. Lyons: S. Gryphius.

―――― (1549) *Aliquot Opera . . . Galeni*. Paris: J. Dupuy.

Funk H (2016) A Little Known Mid-16th Century Description of the Production of English Ale by John Caius. In *Brewery History* 165: 19–29.

―――― (2017) John Caius's Contributions to Conrad Gessner's *Historia Animalium* and 'Historia Plantarum': A Survey With Commentaries. In *Archives of Natural History* 44.2.

―――― (forthcoming) Thomas Penny and Conrad Gessner: A Revision of Some Long-established Chronological Particulars. In *Archives of Natural History*.

Gabel JB (1968) *John Caius. De pronunciatione graecae et latinae linguae cum scriptione nova libellus (1574). A Facsimile and English Translation. Leeds Texts and Monographs*, n.s. 2. Leeds: The University of Leeds. School of English.

Galen (1502) *Opera omnia*. Venice: B. Benalius.

―――― (1517) *De sanitate tuenda*, tr. T Linacre. Paris: D. Mattheu for G. Hittorp.

―――― (1519) *Methodus medendi*. tr. T Linacre. Paris: D. Mattheu for G. Hittorp.

―――― (1525) *Opera omnia*. Venice: heirs of Aldus.

―――― (1536) *Antidotarius liber. . . . translatus a Josepho Struthio . . . Galeni Astrologiae ad Aphrodiseum liber unus, Galeni De urinis liber unus*. Venice: J. A. Nicolini de Sabio.

―――― (1538) *Opera omnia, ad fidem complurium & perquam vetustorum exemplariorum ita emendata atque restituta, ut nunc primum nata, atque in lucem aedita, uideri possint*. Basle: Cratander.

―――― (1541–1542) *Galeni opera quae extant omnia*. Venice: Giunta.

―――― (1541–1545) *Galeni opera omnia*. Venice: G.Farri and brothers.

―――― (1550) *Aliquot opuscula nunc primum Venetorum opera inventa et excusa*. Lyons: G. Rouille.

―――― (1565) *Galeni opera quae extant omnia*. Venice: Giunta.

Garofalo I (ed) (1986–2000) *Galenus, Anatomicarum administrationum libri qui supersunt novem. Earundem interpretatio Arabica Hunaino Isaaci filio ascripta*. Naples: Istituto Orientale.

―――― (2004) Agostino Gadaldino (1515–1575) et le Galien latin. In Boudon-Millot V and Cobolet G (eds) *Lire les médecins grecs à la Renaissance: aux origines de l'édition médicale: actes du colloque international de Paris, 19–20 septembre 2003*. Paris: Bibliothèque interuniversitaire de médecine: 283–322.

―――― (2009) Il falso commento di Galeno al *de humoribus* e un saggio di edizione del vero. In Garofalo I, Lami A and Roselli A (eds) *Sulla tradizione indiretta dei testi medici greci. Atti del II seminario internazionale di Siena, Certosa di Pontignano 19–20 settembre 2088*. Pisa and Rome: Fabrizio Serra Editore: 201–18.

―――― and Debru A (eds) (2005) *Galien, Les os pour les débutants, L'anatomie des muscles*. Paris: Les Belles Lettres.

―――― (eds) (2008) *Galien, L'anatomie des nerfs, L'anatomie des veines et des artères*. Paris: Les Belles Lettres.

Garrison DH (trans) (2015) *Vesalius: The China Root Epistle. A New Translation and Critical Edition*. Cambridge: Cambridge University Press.

―――― and Hast M (trans) (2014) *Andreas Vesalius: The Fabric of the Human Body*. Basle: Karger.

Gärtner F (2012) Galen Rediscovered – Goulston's Basle Edition. In *History Ireland* 20.3: 8–9.

―――― (ed) (2015) *Galeni de locis affectis. CMG* V 6.1,1. Berlin: W. De Gruyter.

Gessner C (1545) *Bibliotheca universalis*. Zurich: C. Froschover.

―――― (1551–1558) *Historia animalium*. Zurich: C. Froschover.

———— (1553) *Icones animalium quadrupedum viviparorum et oviparorum*. Zurich: C. Froschover.

———— (1555) *Appendix Bibliothecae*. Zurich: C. Froschover.

———— (1559) *The Treasure of Euonymus, Conteyninge the Wonderfull Hid Secretes of Nature, Touching the Most Apte Formes to Prepare and Destyl Medicines, for the Conservation of Health*. London: John Daye.

———— (1560a) *Icones animalium quadrupedum viviparorum et oviparorum*, 2nd edition. Zurich: C. Froschover.

———— (1560b) *Icones avium omnium*, 2nd edition. Zurich: C. Froschover.

———— (1562) *De libris suis epistola*. Zurich: C. Froschover.

———— (1577) *Epistolae medicinales*. Zurich: C. Froschover.

———— (1603) *Historiae animalium liber primus de quadrupedibus viviparis*. Frankfurt: R. Cambierius.

Gillet JFA (1860–1861) *Crato von Crafftheim und seine Freunde. Ein Beitrag zur Kirchengeschichte*. Frankfurt: H.L. Brönner.

Gliozzi G (1972) Brasavola, Antonio. In *DBI* 14: 51–2.

———— (1974) Canano, Giovanni Battista, il Giovane. In *DBI* 17: 714–16.

Grafton AT (2017) A Medical Man Among Ecclesiastical Historians: John Caius, Matthew Parker and the History of Cambridge University. In Manning G and Klestinec C (eds) *Professors, Physicians and Practices in the History of Medicine. Essays in Honor of Nancy Siraisi. Archimedes* 50. n.p.: Springer International: 85–100.

Gransden A (1982) *Historical Writing in England. Vol. II. C. 1307 to the Early Sixteenth Century*. London and Henley: Routledge & Kegan Paul.

Grant JN (1998) *Erasmus, On Praying to God: Collected Works of Erasmus*, vol. 70. Toronto, Buffalo and London: University of Toronto Press: 141–230.

Green MAE (ed) (1872) *Calendar of State Papers, Domestic Series, of the Reigns of Elizabeth and James I, 1580–1625. Addenda*. London: Longman & Sons, Trubner & Sons.

Grell OP (2017) Three Seventeenth-century Manuals on How and Where to Study Medicine. In Grell OP and Cunningham A (eds) *Medicine, Natural Philosophy and Religion in Poist-Reformation Scandinavia*. Abingdon and New York: Routledge: 136–52.

Grendler PF (2002) *The Universities in the Italian Renaissance*. London and Baltimore: Johns Hopkins University Press.

Grierson P (1978) John Caius' Library. In Prichard MJ and Skemp JB (eds) *The Biographical History of Gonville and Caius College*, VII.1. Cambridge: Cambridge University Press: 509–25.

Grigson C (2016) *Menagerie: The History of Exotic Animals in England*. Oxford: Oxford University Press.

Gryllus L (1566) *Oratio de peregrinatione studii medicinalis ergo suscepta*. Prague: G. Melantrich.

Guardasole A (2010) Les marginalia de John Caius au *De compositione medicamentorum secundum locos* de Galien dans l'édition de Bâle (1538) de l'Eton College. In Boudon V, Garzya A, Jouanna J and Roselli A (eds) *Storia della tradizione e edizione dei testi medici greci. Atti dl VI Colloquio internazionale Paris 12–14 aprile 2008*. Naples: M. D'Auria: 337–52.

Guinter J (1536) *Institutionum anatomicarum ex Galeni sententia ad candidatos medicinae libri quatuor*. Paris: S. De Colines.

———— (1539) *Institutionum anatomicarum ex Galeni sententia ad candidatos medicinae libri quatuor. Nunc recens ab ipso auctore &recogniti & aucti*. Basle: Robert Winter.

—— (1571) *De medicina veteri et nova tum cognoscenda tum faciunda commentarii duo*. Basle: Officina Henrichpetrina.

—— and Vesalius A (1538) *Institutionum anatomicarum secundum Galeni sententiam ad candidatos medicinae libri quatuor per Ioannem Guinterium Andernacum medicum AB ANDREA VVESALIO BRUxellensi auctiores & emendatiores redditi*. Venice: D. Bernardinus.

Gundert B (2006) Zu den Quellen der Basler Galen-Ausgabe (1538). In Müller CW, Brockmann C and Brunschön W (eds) *Ärzte und ihre Interpreten. Medizinische Fachtexte der Antike also Forschungsgegenstand der Klassischen Philologie. Fachconferenz zu Ehren von Diethard Nickel*. Munich and Leipzig: K. G. Saur: 81–100.

—— (ed) (2009) *Galeni De symptomatum differentiis. CMG* V 5,1. Berlin: Akademie Verlag.

Gunnoe CD and Shackelford J (2009) Johannes Crato von Krafftheim (1519–1585). Imperial physician, irenicist, and anti-Paracelsian. In Plummer ME and Barnes R (eds) *Ideas and Cultural Margins in Early Modern Germany. Essays in Honor of H. C. Erik Midelfort*. Farnham and Aldershot: Ashgate: 201–16.

Haddon W (1567) *Lucubrationes passim collectae et editae . . . studio et labore Thomae Hatcheri Cantabrigiensis*. London: W. Seres.

Harris CRS (1973) *The Heart and the Vascular System in Ancient Greek Medicine From Alcmaeon to Galen*. Oxford: Clarendon Press.

Hart J (1569) *An Orthographie*. London: William Seres.

Hartlich O (ed) (1923) *Galeni De ptisana, CMG* V 4,1,2. Leipzig and Berlin: B. G. Teubner: LVIII–LXIII, 455–63.

Helm J (2001) Religion and Medicine: Anatomical Education at Wittenberg and Ingoldstadt. In Helm J and Winkelmann A (eds) *Confessions and the Sciences in the Sixteenth Century*. Leiden: Brill: 51–68.

Hiatt A (2004) Stow, Grafton, and 15th-Century Historiography. In Gadd I and Gillespie A (eds) *John Stow (1525–1605) and the Making of the English Past*. London: British Library: 45–56.

Hieronymus F (2005) *Theophrast und Galen – Celsus und Paracelsus. Medizin, Naturphilosophie und Kirchenreform im Basler Buchdruck bis zum dreissigjährigen Krieg*. Basle: Universitätsbibliothek.

Hobson A (1975) The iter italicum of Jean Matal. In Hunt RW (ed) *Studies in the Book Trade in Honour of Graham Pollard*. Oxford: Oxford Bibliographical Society: 33–61.

Hoffmann FL (1856) Ein bibliothekarsches Gutachten, abgegeben im Jahre 1631 von Johann Rhodius. In *Intelligenz-Blatt zum Serapeum, Zeitschrift für Bibliothekwissenschaft, Handschriftenkunde und ältere Literatur* 31,2–5: 10–13, 17–21, 25–28, 33–37.

Houlbrooke RA (1974) *The Letter Book of John Parkhurst, Bishop of Norwich, Compiled During the Years 1571–7*. Norfolk: Norfolk Record Society.

Jackson DF (2011) *The Greek Library of Saints John and Paul (San Zanipolo) at Venice*. Tampa: ACMRS.

Jacoby F (1940) *Die Fragmente der griechischen Historiker, Dritter Teil. Geschichte von Städten und Völkern (Horographie und Ethnographie). A Autoren über verschiedene Städte/Länder*. Leiden: E. J. Brill.

—— (1943) *Die Fragmente der griechischen Historiker, Dritter Teil. Geschichte von Städten und Völkern (Horographie und Ethnographie). Kommentar*. Leiden: E. J. Brill.

Jebb S (ed) (1729) *John Caius. De canibus Britannicis, liber unus. De rariorum animalium et stirpium historia, liber unus. De libris propriis, liber unus*. London: Charles Davis.

Joffe SN (2014) *Andreas Vesalius, the Making, the Madman and the Myth*. Bloomington: AuthorHouse.

Johnston I (2006) *Galen on Diseases and Symptoms*. Cambridge: Cambridge University Press.

Jones PM (1988a) Thomas Lorkyn's Dissections, 1564/5 and 1566/7. In *Transactions of the Cambridge Bibliographical Society* 9.3: 209–29.

Jones WRD (1988b) *William Turner, Tudor Naturalist, Physician and Divine*. London and New York: Routledge.

Jouanna J (1982) Littré, éditeur et traducteur d'Hippocrate. In Roger J (ed) *Actes du Colloque Émile Littré 1801–1881, Paris, 7–9 octobre 1981*. Paris: Éditions Albin Michel: 285–302.

——— (2010) Un Galien oublié: *Caractéristiques propres à Hippocrate* (Stobée, *Anthologie* 4.37.14), avec une nouvelle édition. In Boudon-Millot V, Garzya A, Jouanna J and Roselli A (eds) *Storia della tradizione e edizione dei medici greci. Atti del VI Colloquio internazionale, Paris 12–14 aprile 2008*. Naples: M. D'Auria: 199–229.

Jouanna-Bouchet J (2016) *Scribonius Largus, Compositions médicales*. Paris: Les Belles Lettres.

Jugie M (1931) Nicéphore Calliste. In Vacant A, Mangenot E and Amann É (eds) *Dictionnaire de théologie catholique*, VI. Paris: Librairie Letouzey and Ané: 446–52.

King H (2007) *Midwifery, Obstetrics and the Rise of Gynaecology: Users of a Sixteenth-Century Compendium*. Aldershot: Ashgate.

Kitsch M (2004) Day, George. In *ODNB* 15: 581–2.

Klestinec C (2011) *Theaters of Anatomy: Students, Teachers and Traditions of Dissection in Renaissance Venice*. Baltimore: Johns Hopkins University Press.

Knighton CS (ed) (1998) *Calendar of State Papers Domestic Series of the Reign of Mary I 1553–1558*, revised edition. London: Public Record Office.

——— (2004) Thirlby Thomas. In *ODNB* 54: 251–3.

Kozluk NM (2010) Une mystérieuse éditiion de Galien: les opuscula varia, édités par Théodore Goulston et Thomas Gataker (Londres, 1640). In *Revue d'histoire des textes* n.s. 5: 295–306.

Kudlien F and Durling RJ (eds) (1991) *Galen's Method of Healing. Proceedings of the 1982 Galen Symposium. Studies in Ancient Medicine* 1. Leiden and New York: E. J. Brill.

Kühn KG (ed) (1821–1832) *Claudii Galeni opera omnia*. Leipzig: K. Knobloch.

Kusukawa S (2012) *Picturing the Book of Nature: Image, Text and Argument in Sixteenth-Century Human Anatomy and Medical Biology*. Chicago: Chicago University Press.

Labowsky L (1979) *Bessarion's Library and the Biblioteca Marciana: Six Early Inventories. Sussidi Eruditi 31*. Rome: Edizioni di Storia e Letteratura.

Laguna A (1554) *Epitome omnium rerum et sententiarum, quae annotatu dignae in Commentariis Galeni in Hippocratem extant . . . Cui accessere nonnulla Galeni Enantiomata*. Lyons: G. Rouille.

Lamb ME (2009) The Cooke Sisters: Attitudes Toward Learned Women in the Renaissance. In Beilin EV (ed) *Early Tudor Women Writers*. Farnham and Burlington, VT: Ashgate: 379–98.

Lamoreaux JC (2015) *Hunayn ibn Ishaq on His Galen Translations*. Provo: Brigham Young University Press.

Langslow D (2000) *Medical Latin in the Roman Empire*. Oxford: Oxford University Press.

Laoutaris C (2010) Translation/Historical Writing. In Bick C and Summit J (eds) *The History of British Women's Writing, 1500–1610*. London: Macmillan: 296–327.

Law C (2018) *Contested Reformations in the University of Cambridge c. 1535-84*. Woodbridge: Boydell and Brewer.

Lee S and Wallis P (2004) Owen, George. In *ODNB* 42: 198–9.

Lees CJ (1967) *The Poetry of Walter Haddon*. The Hague and Paris: Mouton.

Legrand E (1885) *Bibliographie hellénique ou description raisonnée des ouvrages publiés par des grecs aux XVe et XVIe siècles*, vols. I–IV. Paris: Ernest Leroux.

Lemon R (ed) (1856) *Calendar of State Papers, Domestic Series, of the Reigns of Edward VI, Mary, Elizabeth, 1547–1580*. London: Longman Brown, Green, Longmans & Roberts.

Leoniceno N (1492) *De Plinii et aliorum in medicina erroribus*. Ferrara: L. de Rubeis and A. de Grassis.

——— (1508) *In libros Galeni e greca in linguam latinam a se translatos*. Venice: J. Pentius de Leucho.

Leu UB (1990) *Conrad Gesner als Theologe: ein Beitrag zur Zürcher Geistesgeschichte des 16. Jahrhunderts*. Bern: P. Lang.

——— (2016a) *Conrad Gessner (1516–1565): Universalgelehrter und Naturforscher der Renaissance*. Zürich: Verlag Neue Züricher Zeitung.

——— (2016b) Conrad Gessners Netzwerk. In Lu UB and Ruoss M (eds) *Facetten eines Universums: Conrad Gessner 1516–1565*. Zürich: Verlag Neue Züricher Zeitung: 61–74.

——— and Ruoss M (eds) (2016) *Facetten eines Universums: Conrad Gessner 1516–1565*. Zürich: Verlag Neue Züricher Zeitung.

Lewis RG (1977) The Linacre Lectureships Subsequent to Their Foundation. In Maddison F, Pelling M and Webster C (eds) *Essays on the Life and Work of Thomas Linacre c. 1460–1524*. Oxford: Clarendon Press: 223–64.

Lind LR (1975) *Studies in Pre-Vesalian Anatomy, Biography, Translations, Documents, Memoirs of the American Philosophical Society*, vol. 104. Philadelphia: American Philosophical Society.

Littré E (ed) (1839–1861) *Oeuvres complètes d'Hippocrate*. Paris: J. B. Baillière.

Loades DM (1991) *The Reign of Mary Tudor: Politics, Government and Religion in England, 1553–58*, 2nd edition. London and New York: Longman.

Lonie IM (1975) The Paradoxical Text *On the Heart*. In *Medical History* 17: 1–15, 136–53.

——— (1985) The 'Paris Hippocratics': Teaching and Research in Paris in the Second Half of the Sixteenth Century. In Wear A, French RK and Lonie IM (eds) *The Medical Renaissance of the Sixteenth Century*. Cambridge: Cambridge University Press: 155–74.

Louthan H (1994) *Johannis Crato and the Austrian Habsburgs: Reforming a Counter-Reform Court*. Princeton, NJ: Princeton Theological Seminary.

Lowry MJC (1974–1975) Two Great Venetian Libraries. In *Bulletin of the John Rylands Library* 57: 128–66.

Luce TJ (1977) *Livy: The Composition of His History*. Princeton: Princeton University Press.

Lycosthenes C and Simler J (eds) (1555) *Epitome Bibliothecae Conradi Gesneri*. Zurich: C. Froschover.

Lyons MC (ed) (1969) *Galen on the Parts of Medicine, on Cohesive Causes, on Regimen in Acute Diseases in Accordance With the Theories of Hippocrates. CMG Supplementum Orientale 2*. Berlin: Akademie Verlag.

Maclean I (1999) Interpreting the De libris propriis. In Baldi M and Canziani G (eds) *Girolamo Cardano: le opere, le fonti, la vita*. Milan: FrancoAngeli: 13–33.

——— (2002) *Logic, Signs and Nature in the Renaissance*. Cambridge: Cambridge University Press.

────── (2004) *De libris propriis: The Editions of 1544, 1550, 1557, 1562 With Sup-plementary Material*. Milan: FrancoAngeli.

MacMahon L (2004) Mont, Christopher. In *ODNB* 38: 687–8.

Madan F (1905) *A Summary Catalogue of Western Manuscripts in the Bodleian Library at Oxford*, vol. 5. Oxford: Clarendon Press.

Maddison F (2004) Greaves, John. In *ODNB* 23: 496–7.

──────, Pelling M and Webster C (eds) (1977) *Essays on the Life and Work of Thomas Linacre c. 1460–1524*. Oxford: Clarendon Press.

Magnusson L (2004) Bacon, Anne. In *ODNB* 3: 117–9.

Manetti D and Roselli A (1994a) Il ruolo della tradizione nei libri chirurgici di Celso. In Mudry G and Sabbah G (eds) *La médecine de Celse. Aspects historiques, scien-tifiques et littéraires. Mémoires du Centre Jean Palerne* 13. Saint-Etienne: Publica-tions de l'Université de Saint-Étienne: 103–22.

────── (1994b) Galeno commentatore di Ippocrate. In *Aufstieg und Niedergang der römischen Welt*, II,37,2. Berlin: De Gruyter: 1529–635.

Marchetti V, De Ferrari V and Mutini C (1973) Calcagnini, Celio. In *DBI* 16: 492–8.

Mariani P (1995) Johann Rhode. In Minelli A (ed) *L'Orto botanico di Padova -1545–1595*. Padua: Marsilio: 71–2.

Marra P (1966) Galeno Del movimento del torace e del polmone, traduzione e com-mento. In *Medicina nei Secoli* 34: 38–43.

Marshall P (2017) Settlement Patterns. In Milton A (ed) *The Oxford History of Angli-canism. Volume 1: Reformation and Identity, c. 1529–1662*. Oxford: Oxford Uni-versity Press: 45–59.

Martin CT and Davies RA (2004) Butts, Sir William. In *ODNB* 9: 278–9.

Martius H (1568) *Noni medici clarissimi de omnium morborum curatione*. Stras-bourg: J. Rihel.

Märtl C, Kaiser C and Ricklin T (eds) (2013) *"Inter graecos latinissimus, inter lati-nos graecissimus": Bessarion zwischen den Kulturen*. Berlin: W. De Gruyter.

Marx F (ed) (1915) *A Cornelii Celsi quae supersunt*. Berlin and Leipzig: Teubner.

Massa N (1536) *Liber introductorius anatomiae*. Venice: F. Bindoni and M. Pasini.

────── (1550) *Epistolae medicinales et philosophicae*. Venice: F. Bindoni and M. Pasini.

McCallum-Barry C (2017) Learned Women of the Renaissance and Early Modern England: The Relevance of Their Scholarship. In Wykes R and Hall E (eds) *Women Classical Scholars: Unsealing the Fountain From the Renaissance to Jacqueline de Romilly*. Oxford: Oxford University Press: 29–47.

McCullough D (2017) The Church of England and International Protestantism, 1530–1570. In Milton A (ed) *The Oxford History of Anglicanism: Volume 1. Ref-ormation and Identity, c. 1529–1662*. Oxford: Oxford University Press: 316–32.

McGrath P (1967) *Papists and Puritans Under Elizabeth I*. London: Blandford Press.

McNair A (1969) Why Is the Doctor in 'The Merry Wives of Windsor' Called Caius? In *Medical History* 13: 311–39.

Mei M (ed) (2005) *Collectio thesauri: dalle Marche tesori nascosti di un collezion-ismo illustre*. Florence: Edifir.

Mewaldt J (ed) (1915) *Galeni De comate secundum Hippocratem, CMG* V,9,2. Berlin and Leipzig: B. G. Teubner: xv, 181–94.

Mioni E (1981) Cipelli, Giovanni Battista. In *DBI* 25: 698–702.

Modona L (1889) *Catalogo dei manoscritti ebraici della Biblioteca della r. Univer-sità di Bologna:* Bologna: Biblioteca universitaria.

Mondino de' Liuzzi (1992) *Anothomia*. Bologna: Istituto per la Storia dell'università di Bologna.

Mondrain B (1997) Éditer et traduire les médecins grecs au XVIe siècle: L'exemple de Janus Cornarius. In Jacquart D (ed) *Les voies de la science grecque. Études sur la transmission des textes de l'Antiquité au dix-neuvième siècle*. Geneva: Droz: 391–417.

——— (2017) Le Prorrhétique II dans les traductions de la Collection Hippocratique à la Renaissance. Le traivail éditorial de Marcus Fabius Calvus. In *Galenos* 11: 247–65.

Monfort M-L (2000) L'histoire moderne du fragment hippocratique *Des Remèdes*. In *Revue des Etudes Anciennes* 102: 361–77.

——— (2016) *Janus Cornarius et la redécouverte d'Hippocrate à la Renaissance*. Turnhout: Brepols.

Moore N (1918) *The History of St Bartholomew's Hospital*. London: C. Arthur Pearson.

Morgan V (2004) *A History of the University of Cambridge. Volume II: 1546–1750*. Cambridge: Cambridge University Press.

Muccillo M (1986) Da Monte, Giambattista. In *DBI* 32: 366–7.

Mudry P (1982) *La préface du De medicina de Celse. Texte, traduction et commentaire*. Rome: Institut Suisse de Rome.

Mugnai Carrara D (1991) *La biblioteca di Nicolò Leoniceno: tra Aristotele e Galeno cultura e libri di un medico umanista*. Florence: L.S. Olschki.

Munk W (1878) *The Roll of the Royal College of Physicians of London: Comprising Biographical Sketches of All the Eminent Physicians Whose Names Are Recorded in the Annals. Vol. I 1518 to 1700, ed. 2*. London: The Royal College of Physicians.

Naudé G (1667) *Epistolae*. Geneva: J. H. Widerhold.

Newcombe DG (2004) John Skip. In *ODNB* 50: 874–5.

Nickson T (2005) Moral Edification at Gonville and Caius College, Cambridge. In *Architectural History* 48: 49–68.

Niedermann M and Liechtenhan E (eds) (1968) *Marcellus, De medicamentis liber, Corpus Medicorum Latinorum* V. Berlin: Akademie Verlag.

Nutton V (ed) (1979) *Galen, On Prognosis: Text, Translation, Commentary, CMG* V.8.1. Berlin: Akademie Verlag.

——— (1985a) Conrad Gesner and the English Naturalists. In *Medical History* 29: 93–7.

——— (1985b) Harvey, Goulston and Galen. In *Koroth* 8: 112–22.

——— (1987a) *John Caius and the Manuscripts of Galen: Proceedings of the Cambridge Philological Society, Supplementary*, vol. 13. Cambridge: The Cambridge Philological Society.

——— (1987b) "Qui magni Galeni doctrinam in re medica primus revocavit" Matteo Corti und der Galenismus im medizinischen Unterricht der Renaissance. In Keil G, Moeller B and Trusen W (eds) *Der Humanismus und die oberen Fakultäten, Mitteilungen XIV der Kommission für Humanismusforschung*. Weinheim: VDA: 173–84.

——— (1990) The Anatomy of the Soul in Early Renaissance Medicine. In Dunstan G (ed) *The Human Embryo*. Exeter: University of Exeter Press: 136–57.

——— (1998) An Early Reader of Vesalius' *Fabrica*. In *Vesalius* 3: 73–4.

——— (ed) (1999) *Galen, on My Own Opinions: Text, Translation and Commentary, CMG* V.3.2. Berlin: Akademie Verlag.

——— (2002) In Defence of Kühn. In Nutton V (ed.) *The Unknown Galen*. In *Bulletin of the Institute of Classical Studies, Supplement* 77: 1–7.

——— (2004a) Caius, John (1510–1573). In *ODNB* 9: 480–2.

——— (2004b) Goulston, Theodore (1575–1632). In *ODNB* 23: 83–4.

——— (2004c) Linacre, Thomas (c. 1460–1424). In *ODNB*. 33: 803–6.

——— (ed and trans) (2008a) *Girolamo Mercuriale, De arte gymnastica*. Florence: Leo S.Olschki.

——— (2008b) The Fortunes of Galen. In Hankinson RJ (ed) *The Cambridge Companion to Galen*. Cambridge: Cambridge University Press: 355–90.

——— (2009) Biographical Accounts of Galen, 1340–1660. In Rütten T (ed) *Geschichte der Medizingeschichtsschreibung. Historiographie unter dem Diktat literarischer Gattungen von der Antike bis zur Aufklärung*. Remscheid: Gardez! Verlag: 201–32.

——— (2011) Padua, Religion and English Medicine in the Sixteenth Century. In Ferretto S, Gori P and Rinaldi M (eds) *Libertas philosophandi in naturalibus. Libertà di ricerca e criteri di regolamentazione istituzionale tra '500 e '700*. Padua: CLEUP: 163–76.

——— (2013) *Ancient Medicine*, 2nd edition. London: Routledge.

——— (2017a) *Johann Guinter and Andreas Vesalius, Principles of Anatomy According to the Opinion of Galen*. London: Routledge.

——— (2017b) John Caius, Historian. In Manning G and Klestinec C (eds) *Professors, and Practices in the History of Medicine: Essays in Honor of Nancy Siraisi. Archimedes*, vol. 50. N.p.: Springer International: 69–84.

——— (2018): 1538, A Year of Vesalian Innovation. In *The Journal of Medieval and Early Modern Studies* 48: 42–60.

O'Malley CD (1955) The Relations of John Caius With Andreas Vesalius and Some Incidental Remarks on the Giunta Galen and on Thomas Geminus. In *Journal of the History of Medicine and Allied Sciences* 10: 147–72.

——— (1961) *Thomas Bartholin, on the Burning of His Library and on Medical Travel*. Lawrence: University of Kansas Libraries.

——— (1964) *Andreas Vesalius of Brussels (1514–1564)*. Berkeley and London: University of California Press.

——— (1965) *English Medical Humanists: Thomas Linacre and John Caius*. Lawrence: University of Kansas Press.

Ongaro G (1981) La medicina nello Studio di Padova e nel Veneto. In Folena G (ed) *Storia della cultura veneta. Volume III: Dal primo Quattrocento al concilio di Trento*. Vicenza: Neri Pozza Editore, Part 3: 75–134.

——— (1994) L'insegnamento clinico di Giovan Battista da Monte (1489–1551): una revisione critica. In *Physis. Rivista internazionale di storia della scienza*, n.s. 31: 358–69.

Ortoleva V (1992) *Disticha Catonis in Graecum Translata*. Rome: Edizioni dell' Ateneo.

Owen H (1825) *A History of Shrewsbury*. Shrewsbury: Harding, Lepard and Co.

Pabel HM (1997) *Conversing With God: Prayer in Erasmus' Pastoral Writings*. Toronto and Buffalo: University of Toronto Press.

Page W (ed) (1911) *A History of the County of Somerset*, vol. 2. London: Constable & Co.

Palmer RJ (1981) Nicolò Massa, His Family and His Fortune. In *Medical History* 25: 385–410.

——— (1983) *The Studio of Venice and Its Graduates in the Sixteenth Century*. Padua: Lint.

Pastore A (1998) Gadaldino, agostino. In *DBI* 51: 128–31.

Pellegrin E (1955) *La bibliothèque des Viscontis et des Sforza ducs de Milan au XVᵉ siècle*. Paris: CNRS.

Perosa A (1980) Codici di Galeno postillati dal Poliziano. In Branca V (ed) *Umanesimo e Rinascimento. Studi in onore di P. O. Kristeller*. Florence: Olschki: 1–33.

Petit C (ed) (2009) *Galien. Tome III: Le médecin*. Paris: Les Belles Lettres.

Pettigrew THJ (2007) *Shakespeare and the Practice of Physic: Medical Narratives on the Early Modern English Stage*. Newark: University of Delaware Press.

Pietrobelli A (2013) Une nouvelle copie d'impression de l'Aldine de Galien: le *Guelf-erbytanus Gud. gr.* 11 (= 4198). In *Galenos* 7: 137–49.

———— (forthcoming 1) Peut-on retrouver des manuscrits perdus? Les *marginalia* de Caius et de Scaliger dans leur édition imprimée de Galien. In Ieraci Bio AM, Raiola T and Roselli A (eds) *Actes du VIIe Colloque international sur l'ecdotique des textes médicaux grecs (Procida, 11–13 juin 2013)*.

———— (forthcoming 2) *Ope codicum, ope ingenii?* A la recherche des sources de l'érudition galénique de Janus Cornarius. In La Charité C (ed) *Actes du colloque international 'La réception de Galien à l'époque de Rabelais (Montreal 1 and 2 April 2014)*.

Piovan F (1988) *Per la biografia di Lazzaro Bonamico: ricerche sul periodo dell'insegnamento padovano (1530–1552) Contributi alla storia dell'Università di Padova* 17. Trieste: LINT.

Pitseus J. (1619) *Relationes historicae de rebus Anglicis*. Paris: R. Thierry and S. Cramoisy.

Platt FJ (2004) James, John. In *ODNB* 29: 714–16.

Plomer HR (1926–1927) The 1574 Edition of Dr John Caius's *De Antiquitate Cante-brigiensis Academiae libri* duo. In *The Library*, ser 4.8: 252–68.

Pollard AF and Bakewell S (2004) Wendy, Thomas. In *ODNB* 59: 108.

Pollard AF and Wallis P (2004) Wotton, Edward. In *ODNB* 60: 373–4.

Porter HC (1958) *Reformation and Reaction in Tudor Cambridge*. Cambridge: Cambridge University Press.

Potter P (1998) The *Editiones Principes* of Galen and Hippocrates and Their Relationship. In Fischer KD, Nickel D and Potter P (eds) *Text and Tradition*. Leiden, Boston and Cologne: Brill: 243–61.

———— (2010) *Hippocrates*, vol. 9. London and Cambridge, MA: Heinemann.

Powell JGF (ed) (1995) *Cicero the Philosopher: Twelve Papers*. Oxford: Clarendon Press.

Pratensis J (1527) *De pariente et partu*. Cologne: H. Fuchs.

Priesner P (1997) Münster, Sebastian. In *Neue Deutsche Biographie*, vol. 18. Berlin: Duncker & Humblot: 539–41.

Priestland P (2004) Russell, Elizabeth. In *ODNB* 48: 235–6.

Putter A (2003) King Arthur at Oxbridge: Nicholas Cantelupe, Geoffrey of Monmouth and Cambridge's Arthurian Foundation Myth. In *Medium Aevum* 72: 63–81.

Raeder H (ed) (1928–1929) *Oribasii Collectionum medicarum reliquiae, CMG* VI,1,1–2. Berlin and Leipzig: Teubner.

Raiola T (2015) *Nel tempo di una vita. Studi sull'autobiografia in Galeno*. Pisa and Rome: Fabrizio Serra Editore.

Raugei AM (2001) *Gian Vincenzo Pinelli et Claude Dupuy. Une correspondance entre deux humanistes*. Florence: Olschki.

Raven CE (1947) *The English Naturalists*. Cambridge: Cambridge University Press.

Reed AW (1925–1926) John Clement and His Books. In *The Library*, ser. 4, 6: 329–39.

Rex R (1990–1991) Thomas Vavasour. In *Recusant History* 20: 436–54.

———— (2004a) Bullock, George. In *ODNB* 8: 641–2.

———— (2004b) Vavasour, Thomas. In *ODNB* 56, 225–6.

Reynolds EE (1960) *Margaret Roper: Eldest Daughter of Sir Thomas More*. London: Burns and Oates.

Rhodius J (1639) *De acia dissertatio ad Cornelii Celsi mentem.* Padua: P. Frambotto.

———— (ed) (1655) *Scribonii Largi Compositiones medicae cum notis.* Padua: P. Frambotto.

———— (1672) *De acia dissertatio ad Cornelii Celsi mentem. . . . Accedit de ponderibus et mensuris ejusdem autoris dissertatio, & vita Celsi.* Copenhagen: Godicchenius.

Rocca J (2003) *Galen on the Brain: Anatomical Knowledge and Physiological Speculation in the Second Century AD.* Leiden: Brill.

———— (2008) Anatomy. In Hankinson RJ (ed) *The Cambridge Companion to Galen.* Cambridge: Cambridge University Press: 242–62.

Rosa P (1999) Note sulle'edizioni a stampa del *De motu musculorum* di Galeno. In Garzya A and Jouanna J (eds) *I testi medici greci. Tradizione e ecdotica.* Naples: M. D'Auria: 481–91.

———— (2009) *Galenus De motu musculorum.* Pisa and Rome: Fabrizio Serra.

Rotondò A (1969) Bocchi, Achille. In *DBI* 11: 67–70.

Santing K (2010) Pieter van Foreest and the Acquisition and Travelling of Medical Knowledge in the Sixteenth Century. In Grell OP, Cunningham A and Arrizabalaga J (eds) *Centres of Medical Excellence? Medical Travel and Education in Europe, 1500–1789.* Farnham and Burlington, VT: Ashgate: 49–70.

Savino C (2009) Dare ordine a Galeno. L'edizione di Giovanni Battista Rasario (1562–1563). In Garofalo I, Lami A and Roselli A (eds) *Sulla tradizione indiretta dei testi medici greci. Atti del II seminario internazionale di Siena, Certosa di Pontignano 19–20 settembre 2008.* Pisa and Rome: Fabrizio Serra Editore: 187–200.

Schmitt CB (1974) The University of Pisa in the Renaissance. In *History of Universities* 3: 3–17.

———— (1989) *Reappraisals in Renaissance Thought.* London: Variorum Reprints.

Schoeck RJ (1949) Two Notes on Margaret Giggs. In *Notes and Queries* 194: 532–3.

Schoene H (1924) Hippokrates Περὶ φαρμάκων. In *Rheinisches Museum* 73: 434–48.

———— (1932–1933) Galens Schrift über die Siebenmonatskinder. Iin *Quellen und Studien zur Geschichte d er Naturwissenschaften und der Medizin* 3: 120–38.

Scholz L (ed) (1591–1611) *Johannis Cratonis et aliorum medicorum consilia et epistulae.* Frankfurt: Wechel.

———— (ed) (1610) *Epistolae philosophicae medicinales ac chymicae a summis nostrae aetatis philosophis ac medicis exaratae.* Hanau: Wechel, Heirs of J. Aubry.

Schrenk P (1989) Byzantine Evidence for Galen's *On Medical Experience.* In *Byzantinische Zeitschrift* 82: 251–9.

Schupbach W (1982) *The Paradox of Rembrandt's 'Anatomy of Dr. Tulp', Medical History, Supplement 2.* London: The Wellcome Institute.

Sconocchia S (ed) (1983) *Scribonius Largus, Compositiones.* Leipzig: Teubner.

Serbat G (ed) (1995) *Celse. De la médecine.* Paris: Les Belles Lettres.

Serrai A (1990) *Conrad Gesner.* Rome: Bulzoni.

Shalev Z (2005) The Travel Diaries of John Greaves. In Hamilton A, Van den Boogert MH and Westerweel B (eds) *The Republic of Letters and the Levant: Intersections, Yearbook for Early Modern Studies*, vol. 5. Leiden: Brill: 77–102.

Shaw A (2003) *The Compendium Compertorium and the Making of the Suppression Act of 1536*, Ph.D. thesis, University of Warwick.

Shuger D (2009) A Protesting Catholic Puritan in Elizabethan England. In *The Journal of British Studies* 48: 587–630.

Simler J (1566) *Vita clarissimi philosophi et medici excellentissimi Conradi Gesneri Tigurini, conscripta à Josia Simlero Tigurino. Item Epistola Gesneri, de libris a se editis. . . .* Zurich: C. Froschover.

Simon M (ed) (1906) *Sieben Bücher Anatomie des Galen.* Leipzig: J. C. Hinrichs'sche Buchhandlung.

Singer C and Rabin C (1946) *A Prelude to Modern Science: Being a Discussion of the History, Sources and Circumstances of the 'Tabulae Anatomicae Sex' of Vesalius.* Cambridge: Cambridge University Press.

Singkeler S (1537) *Medicorum schola, hoc est, Claudii Galeni Isagoge.* Basle: T. Platter and B. Lasius.

Siraisi NG (1990) *Medieval and Early Renaissance Medicine: An Introduction to Knowledge and Practice.* Chicago: Chicago University Press.

——— (1997) *The Clock and the Mirror: Girolamo Cardano and Renaissance Medicin.* Princeton: Princeton University Press.

Skaarup BO (2015) *Anatomy and Anatomists in Early Modern Spain.* Farnham and Burlington, VT: Ashgate.

Skoda F (1988) *Médecine antique et métaphore: Le vocabulaire de l'anatomie et de la pathologie en grec ancien.* Paris: Peeters/Selaf.

Smith MHH (1974) Some Humanist Libraries in Early Tudor Cambridge. In *The Sixteenth Century Journal* 5.1: 18–34.

Smith T (1568a) *De recta et emendata linguae graecae pronuntiatione.* Paris: R. Estienne.

——— (1568b) *De recta et emendata linguae Anglicae scriptione.* Paris: R. Estienne.

Smith WD (1979) *The Hippocratic Tradition.* Ithaca: Cornell University Press.

Snorrason E (1965) *Danskeren Johan Rhode: i det 17. århundredes.* Padua and Copenhagen: Mönlycke.

Sollerius JB, Pinius J, Cuperus G and Boschius P (1867) *Acta Sanctorum, August, Part II.* Paris and Rome: V. Palmé.

Sowerby TA (2010) *Renaissance and Reform in Tudor England: The Careers of Sir Richard Morison.* Oxford: Oxford University Press.

Spach I (1597) *Gynaeciorum sive de mulierum tum communibus, tum gravidarum, parientium, et puerperarum affectibus et morbis, libri Graecorum, Arabum, Latinorum veterum et recentium quotquot extant.* Strasbourg: L. Zetzner.

Steinmann M (1969) Aus dem Briefwechsel der Basler Druckers Johann Oporinus. In *Basler Zeitschrift für Geschichte und Altertumskunde* 59: 103–203.

Stevenson J (ed) (1866) *Calendar of State Papers, Foreign Series, of the Reign of Queen Elizabeth Preserved in the State Paper Department of Her Majesty's Public Record Office, Volume 4, 1561–1562.* London: Longman Green.

Stevenson J (2009) Mildred Cecil, Lady Burleigh: Poetry, Politics and Protestantism. In Beilin EV (ed) *Early Tudor Women Writers.* Farnham and Burlington, VT: Ashgate: 427–49.

Stoner J (1931) *The Book of My Life (De vita propria Liber) by Jerome Cardan.* London and Toronto: J. M. Dent.

Strype J (1821) *The Life of the Learned Sir John Cheke.* Oxford: Clarendon Press.

Sylvius J (1556) *In Hippocratis et Galeni physiologicae partem anatomicam isagoge.* Basle: J. Derbilley.

Tavoni MG (1991) Il patrimonio bibliografico a stampa della biblioteca del S: Salvatore. In Tavoni MG and Zani G (eds) *Giovanni Grisostomo Trombelli (1697–1780) e i Canonici Regolari del SS.* Modena: Mucchi: 71–87.

Thorpe SM (1982) Marrow, Thomas. In Bindoff ST (ed) *The History of Parliament: The House of Commons 1509–1558*, vol. 2. London: Secker and Warburg: 573–4.

Tomasini GF (1639) *Bibliothecae Patavinae publicae et privatae*. Udine: N. Schiratto.

———— (1654) *Gymnasium Patavinum*. Udine: N. Schiratto.

Toselli AF (ed) (2003) *La Biblioteca pubblica di Ferrara: 250 anni di libri e lettori: 1753–2003*. Ferrara: Centro stampa Comune di Ferrara.

Traister BH (2004) 'Note Her a Little Farther': Doctors and Healers in the Drama of Shakespeare. In Moss S and Peterson KL (eds) *Disease, Diagnosis and Cure on the Early Modern Stage*. Aldershot: Ashgate: 43–4.

———— (2015) A French Physician in an English Community. In Gajowski E and Rackin P (eds) *The Merry Wives of Windsor: New Critical Essays*. London and New York: Routledge: 121–7.

Van Foreest P (1589–1609) *Observationum et curationum medicalium libri*. Leiden: Plantin for F. Raphelengius.

Venn J (ed) (1904) *The Annals of Gonville and Caius College Cambridge by John Caius*. Cambridge: Cambridge Antiquarian Society.

———— (1912) John Caius. In Roberts ES (ed) *The Works of John Caius, MD*. Cambridge: Cambridge University Press: 1–78.

———— and Venn JA (1922) *Alumni Cantabrigienses, a Biographical List of All Known Students, Graduates and Holders of Office at the University of Cambridge, From the Earliest Times to 1900. Part 1. From the Earliest Times to 1751*. Cambridge: Cambridge University Press.

Vesalius A (1538) *Tabulae Anatomicae Sex*. Venice: B. Vitalis.

———— (1543) *De humani corporis fabrica*. Basle: J. Oporinus.

———— (1555) *De humani corporis fabrica*, 2nd edition. Basle: J. Oporinus.

———— (1564) *Anatomicarum Gabrielis Falloppii Observationum Examen*. Venice: F. de Franciscis.

Virgoe R (1982) Steward, Augustine. In Bindoff ST (ed) *The History of Parliament: The House of Commons 1509–1558*, vol. 3. London: Secker and Warburg: 383–5.

Von Staden H (1989) *Herophilus: The Art of Medicine in Hellenistic Alexandria*. Cambridge: Cambridge University Press.

———— (2017) 'A Woman Does Not Become Ambidextrous'. Galen and the Culture of Scientific Commentary. In Gibson RK and Kraus CS (eds) *The Classical Commentary: Histories, Practices, Theory, Mnemosyne*, Supplement 232. Boston and Leiden: Brill: 109–39.

Wallis P (2004) Clement, John. In *ODNB* 12: 20–2.

Walsham A (1999) *Church Papists: Catholicism, Conformity and Confessional Polemic in Early Modern England*. Woodbridge: The Boydell Press.

———— (2014) *Catholic Reformation in Protestant Britain*. Farnham and Burlington: Ashgate.

Walzer R (1935) Galens Schrift über die Siebenmonatskinder. In *Rivista di Studi Orientali* 15: 323–57.

———— (1944) *Galen on Medical Experience*. Oxford: Clarendon Press.

———— and Frede M (1985) *Three Treatises on the Nature of Science*. Indianapolis: Hackett Publishing Company.

Waquet F (2001) *Latin or the Empire of a Sign, From the Sixteenth to the Twentieth Centuries*. London and New York: Verso.

Wear A (1981) Galen in the Renaissance. In Nutton V (ed) *Galen: Problems and Prospects*. London: Wellcome Institute for the History of Medicine: 229–62.

Welti ME (1964) *Der Basler Buchdruck und Britannien. Die Rezeption britischen Gedankenguts in den Basler Pressen von den Anfängen bis zum Beginn des 17. Jahrhunderts*. Basle: Helbing & Lichtenhan.

Wenkebach E (1925) *John Clement, ein englischer Humanist und Arzt des sechzehnten Jahrhunderts. Ein Lebensbild in Umrissen. Studien zur Geschichte der Medizine*, vol. 18. Leipzig: J. A. Barth.

———— (1933) Textkritische Beiträge zu Galens Protreptikosfragment. In *Sudhoffs Archiv für Geschichte der Medizin* 26: 205–52.

Westenberger J (ed.) (1914) *Galeni De diaeta Hippocratis in morbis acutis. CMG* V,9,1. Leipzig and Berlin: B.G. Teubner: XXXIX–XLVI: 367–92.

White FV (2004) Fryer, John. In *ODNB* 21: 119.

Withington ET (1928) *Hippocrates*, vol. 3. London and Cambridge, MA: Heinemann.

Woolfson J (1997) John Claymond, Pliny the Elder, and the Early History of Corpus Christi College, Oxford. In *English Historical Review* 112: 882–903.

———— (1998) *Padua and the Tudors. English Students in Italy 1485–1603*. Cambridge: James Clarke & Co. Ltd.

———— (2004) Sir Richard Morison. In *ODNB* 39: 187–90.

Worm O (1751) *Olai Wormii et ad eum doctorum virorum epistulae*. Copenhagen: n.p.

Wuttke W (1974) *Otto Sperlings Animadversiones in Scribonium et notas Johannis Rhodii. Einleitung und Edition*. Ph.D. Diss., Tübingen.

Wykes A (1969) *Doctor Cardano, Physician Extraordinary*. London: Friedrich Muller.

Zwinger T (1565) *Theatrum vitae humanae*, 19 vols. Basle: J. Oporinus and A. Froben.

Index